menopause
confidential

menopause
confidential

A Doctor Reveals
the Secrets to Thriving
Through Midlife

Tara Allmen, MD

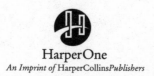

HarperOne
An Imprint of HarperCollinsPublishers

HarperOne

This book contains advice and information relating to healthcare. It should be used to supplement rather than replace the advice of your doctor or another trained health professional. If you know or suspect you have a health problem, it is recommended that you seek your physician's advice before embarking on any medical program or treatment. All efforts have been made to assure the accuracy of the information contained in this book as of the date of publication. This publisher and the author disclaim liability for any medical outcome that may occur as a result of applying the methods suggested in this book.

First Edition

Designed by Paul Barrett

Library of Congress Cataloging-in-Publication Data
Names: Allmen, Tara, author.
Title: Menopause confidential : a doctor reveals the secrets to thriving through
    midlife / Tara Allmen, MD.
Description: First edition. | New York, NY : HarperOne, [2016] | Includes index.
Identifiers: LCCN 2016028325 (print) | LCCN 2016030787 (ebook) |
    ISBN 9780062447265 (hardback) | ISBN 9780062563002 (audio) | ISBN
    9780062447296 (e-book)
Subjects: LCSH: Menopause--Popular works. | Middle-aged women--Health and
    hygiene--Popular works. | BISAC: HEALTH & FITNESS / Women's Health.
    | MEDICAL / Gynecology & Obstetrics. | HEALTH & FITNESS / Healthy
    Living.
Classification: LCC RG186 .A46 2016 (print) | LCC RG186 (ebook) | DDC
    618.1/75--dc23
LC record available at https://lccn.loc.gov/2016028325.

ISBN 9780062447265

16 17 18 19 20   RRD   10 9 8 7 6 5 4 3 2 1

My children would like me to dedicate *Menopause Confidential* to them, which is hilarious because they are barely tweenagers.

So to my smart, funny, and gorgeous Ava and Mark, you were so noisy this past year, you made it practically impossible to write this book. I love you anyway.

I would also like to give a shout-out to my smart, funny, and gorgeous husband, Larry, whom I've had to shout at all year long to help me care for our noisy children. I love you too.

And then there is Sadie, my best dog and favorite furry four-legged daughter, who supported me through many lonely and arduous months by giving me lots of slobbery kisses and loud woofs. I love you the most.

To my smart, funny, and gorgeous parents, Rick and Renée, and my sweet brother, Mark, I wish you were all still here to celebrate with me.

And finally, to all of the women I have had the great honor and privilege of caring for and the many midlife women reading *Menopause Confidential* . . .

Thank you, from the bottom of my heart.

I wouldn't be here without all of you.

CONTENTS

INTRODUCTION

A study says owning a dog makes you ten years
younger. My first thought was to rescue two more,
but I don't want to go through menopause again.

—JOAN RIVERS

WAS THAT . . . ?
   No.
   It couldn't be.
   I'm too young.
   But it sure felt like . . .
   That is how I felt when I experienced my first hot flash at the age of forty-five. For so many of us, bewilderment is followed by denial and then . . . more denial! No woman wants to admit that she is skirting the edges of midlife or maybe is even right in the thick of it.

   At some point in our forties, most of us will begin to notice the inevitable signs of aging as our bodies change in ways for which we are not prepared. While we are pretty good at educating young girls ahead of time about the journey through puberty, and even better at teaching women what to expect when expecting, we get a failing grade when it comes to addressing the changes that occur during perimenopause and menopause. For this reason, many women show up to the conversation basically clueless and without scientifically accurate information. It's no wonder that hitting the perimenopausal and menopausal years throws us for a loop.

You probably did not realize that there is a lot you can easily do to renew your energy, sexual vitality, and good looks. It doesn't have to be all sweaty, sleepless nights; dispiriting weight gain; irritable moods; and a diminished sex life. So don't throw up your hands and accept that you will never feel like yourself again. I am here to be your midlife cheerleader. You are definitely going to get through these difficult times with your health and happiness reinstated.

IT IS A PLEASURE TO MEET YOU

Let me introduce myself. I am a board-certified gynecologist in New York City and a NAMS Certified Menopause Practitioner (NCMP) who specializes in midlife women's health. I see patients ranging from those in the first blush of hot flashes to those deep in the throes of mood swings and brain fog. Most of them feel as though they're having an out-of-body experience. And I get it. Having celebrated my fifty-first birthday recently, it is not just professional for me—it's personal. I know exactly how you feel.

Once we hit menopause, we will be menopausal until the end of our days. Some people refer to the entire period as "postmenopause." This may be a new concept for you, and I know it sounds daunting. But it won't actually be daunting if you know how to deal with the symptoms and protect your health. That last part is especially important. Menopause marks the beginning of a long journey that puts us at higher risk for heart disease, osteoporosis, diabetes, cancer, and other health challenges. So let's not squander valuable time. Instead, join me and learn all about the healthy and productive life that is waiting for you.

HEALTH IS ON THE WAY!

Are you wondering if you will ever feel like your normal self again? My answer is definitely "Yes!" I know there are many books and websites you can read to learn about how to deal with all of your symptoms. I checked most of them out and found the majority to be confusing and not grounded in science. Astonishingly, a lot of information out there is not even provided by an expert in women's health. If I want to learn how to build an airplane or change a carburetor, I most certainly want to learn from the best in that field. Don't you agree? There are, by the way, some excellent and accurate resources that *are* written by experts, and I will reference them at the end of this book.

Most of you will not be able to schlep all the way to New York City to become my patients, but reading *Menopause Confidential* will be like having a fun and informative conversation with me. I am going to address all of your fears and concerns with easy to understand information that is based on scientific evidence. You don't have time to slog through a complicated and lengthy medical treatise. So I am offering you the busy woman's guide to midlife women's health. The following is everything you need to know. And I promise to clear up all the confusing information about perimenopause and menopause.

Menopause Confidential, though, is far more than just a compendium of advice for dealing with hot flashes and midlife muffin top. It is a head-to-toe and everything-in-between guide to living a healthy life. I want you to not only start feeling and looking better right now, but also make great choices for your health in the future. How often do you need to get a Pap? What about mammograms and colonoscopies? How can you guard against heart disease, the number *one* killer of women in the United States? What is the secret to losing weight in midlife? There's a lot of confusion out there, and even the stuff that is on-target can be overwhelming.

So let's get this show on the road and have some fun learning and getting smarter by the minute.

MY STORY

Many women do not like to reveal their age. I am not one of those women. When I turned fifty years young, I shouted it from the rooftops. I was born December 18, 1964, on the small island of Manhattan and raised on a crazy block in the East Village called St. Marks Place. My parents, Rick and Renée, bought apartment buildings in this area in the 1960s and 1970s, a time when the neighborhood was gritty, dangerous, and filled with people doing drugs and living on the streets. As a kid, it was my job to sweep up the hallways and front stoops of my parents' buildings, so I got to see firsthand the harsh effects of taking drugs. I like to say that kids often rebel against the environment they are raised in, and I was no exception. I rebelled against the bad choices taking place all around my neighborhood. Instead of doing drugs, I stayed in my room and did my homework. I loved school, and I loved getting good grades. I went to a small Jewish elementary school just three blocks away from our apartment building in the East Village. My brother, Mark, and I had to walk through the notorious Tompkins Square Park, teeming with addicts and homeless people, in order to get there.

Mark had kidney disease, and many of my childhood hours were spent visiting him in the hospital. I can still remember the exciting wheelchair races we had in the hospital hallways. Seeing medicine at work up close and personal at such an early age really influenced my career choice. There was no doubt in my mind that I would one day become a doctor. I had already decided by the time I was six years old. My brother grew up to be a lawyer. My mother, the landlord, used to joke that she wished one of us had chosen to become a plumber, because plumbers were so expensive. One could make the argument that I did indeed grow up to become a plumber of sorts . . . for women!

I spent the next four years at the prestigious Stuyvesant High School located just six blocks from home. I never really made it out of the East Village until it was time to go to college. I attended Johns Hopkins University as a premed student. Next came medical school at the State University of New York at Stony Brook on Long Island. When it was time to choose a residency, I selected the University of California, San Francisco, not only because it had an excellent program, but also because it was time for me to experience somewhere besides New York City. To this day, I consider myself a sister of San Francisco.

Early in my career, I practiced both obstetrics and gynecology. I really loved delivering babies, performing surgery, and being a partner in the lives of women going through both major and minor health issues. However, at some point in my early thirties, I realized

ssion for taking care of women in their forties and
hough I wasn't quite there yet myself, I felt a real con-
men who were struggling with symptoms that they
had little information about. I decided to change the focus of my
career to midlife women's health.

My decision to stop delivering babies and concentrate on menopause was unusual for an OB-GYN in her thirties. Obstetricians
generally continue to deliver babies until they and their patients
grow older. I was a trailblazer. In 1999, I left my private obstetrical
practice and joined the Center for Menopause, Hormonal Disorders,
and Women's Health in New York City. I have been there ever since.
I also joined the North American Menopause Society (NAMS), the
premier midlife women's health organization dedicated to research
in women's health as well as the ongoing education for both healthcare professionals and women. When your healthcare professional
has earned the prestigious NCMP credential offered only by NAMS,
you can feel confident that you have indeed found someone with
the right expertise to help you through your menopause transition.
I am also very proud of the fact that I have been the president of the
North American Menopause Society Foundation board for the past
three years.

When I first joined the Center for Menopause in New York City,
I had very few patients. My practice grew slowly, largely through
word of mouth. Most women didn't know that a menopause specialist existed. Most women *still* don't know! Women are always
surprised to learn that once they have completed childbearing, it is
time to graduate to a practice that focuses on the needs of women in
midlife. Women are also surprised to learn that not every gynecologist knows everything about menopausal medicine or is passionate

about working with women in transition. Midlife is a complicated and confusing time for most of us. Yet despite the need for experts in the area—and despite the fact that there are about 123 million women between the ages of forty and sixty-five—menopausal medicine is not a large part of the teaching curriculum in OB-GYN residency programs. So it is no surprise that the average OB-GYN does not know much about all the nuances and treatment options needed to help you.

Which is all my way of saying that you have come to the right place.

LET'S GET DOWN TO BUSINESS

The fact that some books on perimenopause and menopause can double as a doorstop may give you the impression that you need to become a midlife health scholar just to get a grip on night sweats. That is simply not true. In the following pages, I'm going to cut to the chase and provide you with all the information you need to understand the changes in your body and how to address them.

I am all about getting the job done thoroughly and efficiently—in every aspect of my life. When I decided it was time to get married and have children, I joined Match.com, an online dating service. Within two weeks, I met the man I would marry, Lawrence Kimmel. I like to joke that he cost me $24.95. Next came our dog, Sadie, followed by our daughter, Ava, and our son, Mark. I gave birth to Ava when I was forty years old and Mark at forty-one and a half. Given my older age when I had kids, my patients often ask whether I had any medical assistance. The truth is that I was very lucky and only needed a little help from my husband.

So go ahead, turn on your air conditioner and settle in for an entertaining and informative read that is sure to change your life for the better. Or your money back. (I'm only kidding about that last part.)

TARA ALLMEN, MD

Physician, wife, mother,
dog lover, philanthropist, and
menopausal woman

CHAPTER 1

Girls Are Made of Sugar and Spice and Everything Nice . . . and That Everything Nice Is Estrogen

After thirty, a body has a mind of its own.

—BETTE MIDLER

I'M ALWAYS SURPRISED TO learn that smart women around the country are still confused about the difference between perimenopause and menopause. Perhaps it's because the two often get lumped together. I get desperate phone calls and e-mails all the time from women asking about symptoms and solutions for both stages of life. Even though they may not know which stage they are officially in, they are worried nonetheless. So let's clear all that up. I am going to devote this chapter to explaining the basics about perimenopause,

menopause, and the hormone shifts that set them in motion. You will never, ever be confused again.

PERIMENOPAUSE VS. MENOPAUSE

Perimenopause, which is the phase leading up to menopause, usually starts in our forties and, on average, lasts from four to eight years. The perimenopausal journey is often heralded by changes in our menstrual cycles. That could mean skipped, more frequent, heavier, or lighter cycles. It could mean just spotting for a while, then the cycles returning to normal again.

Now comes the Oprah aha! moment. Perimenopausal women still *have* menstrual cycles. That means you are still making estrogen and progesterone. And, it is important to note, you can still become pregnant. In fact, after the teenagers, it's the perimenopausal crowd that has the most unintended pregnancies because they think they are no longer fertile. So, perimenopausal ladies, do not throw out your contraceptives yet!

During perimenopause, the monthly conversation between the brain and ovaries is changing because the aging ovaries are less responsive. For that reason, the ovaries don't produce estrogen and progesterone as reliably as they once did. Sometimes they will make too much estrogen, sometimes they will make too little, and sometimes they will make it just right. This sounds a little like the story of Goldilocks and the three bears, but it's more like your local amusement park roller coaster. The perimenopausal body is on a hormonal roller-coaster ride. I love roller coasters, but not when they involve my hormones.

Interestingly, perimenopausal women will experience many of

the same symptoms as menopausal women, such as hot flashes, night sweats, brain fog, sleep problems, fatigue, moodiness, and decreased sexual interest. Those symptoms are due to that hormonal roller-coaster ride. That is why, when talking about relief for perimenopausal symptoms, I like to compare it to getting off the roller coaster and onto a nice and steady tram ride.

Menopause is physiologically very different from perimenopause. The average age of menopause is fifty-one. Some women will transition sooner and some later. However, most women will experience natural menopause between the ages of forty and fifty-eight. Menopause before the age of forty is called premature menopause. Having your ovaries removed surgically is called surgical menopause.

The telltale sign of menopause is no longer having menstrual cycles and, therefore, no longer making estrogen and progesterone from your ovaries. Menopause starts immediately after your last menstrual period. How on earth will you know which is your very last one? Remember that perimenopausal women can skip cycles and then, a few months later, get their period again. So don't label yourself menopausal until you know for sure that you are no longer menstruating. By the way, the formal definition of menopause is when you have not had a menstrual cycle for twelve months in a row.

Some healthcare professionals will measure your FSH level to see if you are in menopause. FSH, or follicle-stimulating hormone, is produced in the brain and increases as you transition through menopause. I rarely measure FSH levels because they can be elevated in *both* perimenopause and menopause, so the test really doesn't provide definitive answers.

A Quick Guide to Perimenopause and Menopause

Perimenopause

» It begins in your 40s
» You're having periods, but they're getting irregular
» You're producing estrogen and progesterone
» You're able to conceive
» It lasts 4 to 8 years

Menopause

» The average age is 51, but the range is 40 to 58
» You have no periods for 12 months in a row
» You're not producing estrogen and progesterone from the ovaries
» It never ends

Now that you have the basic definitions for perimenopause and menopause, which category do you fall into? And does it matter? Isn't a hot flash a hot flash, regardless? In fact, your answer is very important, because perimenopausal women are not menopausal. That sounds so obvious, doesn't it? Yet many healthcare professionals treat these distinct groups similarly when it comes to offering treatment options for symptoms. By the time you finish this book, you will know exactly what the best symptom-relief choices are for you based on your perimenopausal or menopausal status.

YOUR HORMONES, YOURSELF

There's a great lyric from a Joni Mitchell song that says, "Don't it always seem to go, that you don't know what you've got 'til it's gone." That is how I feel about estrogen. We take it completely for granted as younger women, then once we no longer make it, we wish for the days when it was plentiful and doing all the wonderful things for our bodies that it used to do.

Estrogen is a hormone that is primarily made in our ovaries as part of the reproductive process. You probably learned about this in high school, but who among us can remember much of anything from way back then? I think my version of the birds-and-the-bees lecture here will lead you to a better understanding of what is happening to your body now. Let's start at the very beginning, a very good place to start.

At puberty, a fascinating monthly conversation occurs between your brain and ovaries. The goal of the brain is to get one of the eggs nestled inside an ovary to mature and release into the arms of an awaiting sperm. If fertilization occurs and all goes according to plan, the resulting embryo will float down the fallopian tube and land safely inside a soft and fluffy uterine cavity where it will remain for the next nine months and result in a bouncing baby. (By the way, I used to deliver babies. They do not bounce. I have no idea what that expression means or from where it comes. I digress.) During this process, called ovulation, the maturing egg produces estrogen, which, among other duties, helps create the soft lining inside the uterus, giving the embryo a comfortable place to implant and grow.

Your menstrual cycle truly is a cycle. At the beginning, which starts when you are actually having your period, your ovary gears up to recruit an egg. At that time, the egg is mainly producing estrogen. Next, in the middle of your cycle, ovulation occurs. Not only is estrogen helping the chosen egg to ovulate, it is also fluffing up the lining of the uterus in anticipation of a pregnancy.

Once ovulation takes place, you enter the second half of your monthly cycle, and ovarian hormone production shifts to progesterone. Progesterone is mainly in charge of putting the finishing touches on the fluffed-up uterine lining. If no embryo arrives and implants, the uterus sheds its lining. That is called a menstrual period. To your body, it represents a pregnancy failure. Now the brain and the ovaries have to begin their monthly conversation all over again. Another egg is prepared for ovulation, and estrogen and progesterone are back in production, with the hope that the next month's cycle will result in a fertilized egg.

Your Reproductive Hormones: What Does What During the Menstrual Cycle

» Estrogen—advances ovulation and makes the lining of the uterus soft and fluffy
» Progesterone—assists estrogen by stabilizing the soft and fluffy uterine lining
» Testosterone—boosts libido

Estrogen has many other important jobs besides helping to perpetuate the human species. Practically every organ in your body has estrogen receptors, enabling circulating estrogen to get in there and assist with important physiological functions. There are estrogen receptors in the heart, bone, brain, bladder, breast, vagina, colon, and beyond. So you can see why women need estrogen to maintain overall health and wellness. In the absence of estrogen, your body will change in noticeable ways. For instance, there will be a decline in the quality, quantity, and texture of your hair. Your skin will begin to wrinkle and sag. Your nails will weaken, and your vision will worsen. But wait! There's more. Other less obvious changes will occur. Most of you will notice when you begin losing your hair, but few of you will notice that you're getting clogged arteries or losing bone. Without estrogen, we have a lot less of our sugar and spice and everything nice.

Progesterone produced by the ovaries plays a very important role in helping estrogen stabilize the lining of the uterus and support a pregnancy for the first few months. Eventually, the placenta will take over progesterone production. Progesterone is also the hormone that is associated with premenstrual symptoms like irritability, bloating, and fatigue. We really do have to put up with those nuisances, if we want to become pregnant.

Now please pay very close attention, because I am about to shed light on a difficult concept regarding the use of hormone therapy for the treatment of menopausal symptoms. When it comes to the use of progesterone, I want you to understand that progesterone is *not* the hormone that will help you with symptom relief. That is exclusively the job of estrogen. Progesterone has only one purpose in the realm of hormone therapy and that is to protect the uterine lining from abnormal growth as a direct consequence of the estrogen exposure.

So while you may have read about the use of progesterone cream for the treatment of perimenopausal and menopausal symptoms, that is not progesterone's job. Its main duty is to stabilize the uterine lining. If you have had a hysterectomy and therefore do not have a uterus, you do not need progesterone therapy at all. There will be much more on this topic in chapter 16, "Potions, Patches, and Pills, Oh My!"

Testosterone is another hormone made in our ovaries. Yes, even our ovaries must multitask. Testosterone levels rise right before ovulation, which is perfect timing because testosterone is what helps women get "in the mood" just as an egg is ready to be fertilized. Testosterone is also integral to helping us maintain our sense of energy, well-being, and bone strength. After menopause, our ovaries will continue to produce testosterone for a few more years. That explains why women usually don't notice changes in libido until several years *after* the last menstrual period. I will talk more about testosterone and its role in sexual health in chapter 6, "The Vagina Is like Las Vegas, *Baby*!"

THE TRUTH ABOUT AGE

This brings me to my evolving philosophy on aging. I know I am going against the youth-seeking grain when I say this, but I believe that fifty is the new fifty! Having recently passed the half-century mark, I know for sure that it is not the new forty. Women in midlife cannot take ten years off our bodies, nor should we try. However, we can look and feel fantastic at the age we are and, most important, make great strides in maintaining and even improving our health. If not now, when? This is not a rhetorical question. What are you going to do differently to be the best and healthiest you can possibly be as you hit every milestone? In the coming pages, I will reveal *all* the secrets to achieving your goals and much more.

CHAPTER 2

I Am Hot!

I don't have hot flashes. I have short,
private vacations in the tropics.

—ANONYMOUS

WHEN I WAS FORTY-FIVE years old, I went to dinner with my husband and a friend. All of a sudden, I became intensely hot, sweaty, and uncomfortable. The hotter I got, the more agitated I became. Finally, I turned to my husband and asked, "Is it hot in here?" When he said "No," I questioned the obvious: *Could this be a hot flash? Am I going through menopause? I'm way too young!* My husband joked that he knew a good doctor I should see . . . me! Very funny.

If you are a woman in midlife reading this book during the summertime, the answer to the question "Is it hot in here?" is probably "Yes." If it's wintertime and you're still answering "Yes" as you crank up the air-conditioning, read on. This chapter is dedicated to all the women who have ever said to me, "You don't understand how terrible my hot flashes are. I completely soak through my nightgown and sheets." My answer to all of you is that I definitely understand. I am there too, sisters!

THE DREADED—AND PRETTY MUCH UNAVOIDABLE—HOT FLASH

Hot flashes are the most common menopause symptom and the second most common perimenopause symptom. Over 80 percent of women in the United States experience hot flashes. That is a staggering number of *hot* women! Did you know that practically 100 percent of you hot-flashers have done a Google search on the term? That makes "hot flash" the most frequently searched menopause topic on the Internet.

The latest news flash on hot flashes is that they last a lot longer than was formerly thought. The average woman will experience hot flashes for at least seven years, and some will suffer for longer than twenty. I actually do hear from women in their seventies who are surprised and dismayed that they are still flashing. The good news is that you cannot die from a hot flash. You also will not die from the embarrassment of suddenly sweating buckets in the middle of an important work meeting or while making small talk at a party. However, the bad news is that hot flashes can significantly affect your *quality of life.*

What is a hot flash, anyway, and what causes it? The first question is easy to answer. A hot flash is a sudden sensation of heat that usually starts in your upper chest area and then moves to your face.

The usual sequence of events is that you start to feel warm, then hot, and then you begin to flush, which makes you red in the face.

A hot flash can last up to five minutes and is sometimes associated with a fast heart rate, called palpitations, as well as feelings of anxiety. In fact, many women describe feeling like they are having a panic attack right before a hot flash occurs. This panicky feeling is a very scary experience and leads many of you to visit your local emergency room to rule out a heart attack. You might also experience cold chills immediately after a hot flash. That is your body's attempt to regulate its internal temperature and get you back into a comfortable zone. While the concept of having cold chills as a follow-up to a hot flash seems nice, this cool down mechanism can wind up making you feel clammy and sticky. Eventually, your skin temperature will return to normal, but the whole experience could take up to thirty minutes. Who has that kind of time, especially if you're having many hot flashes a day?

THE NIGHT SWEAT NIGHTMARE

Let's not forget about hot flashes' equally annoying cousin, night sweats—which, by the way, also occur during the day. A sweat is really just your body's attempt to cool you down after flashing, and that can happen at any time. While you will definitely feel the hot flash during sleep, you'll really be *awakened* by the sweating part. This will, of course, lead to a less restorative sleep and leave you feeling tired and cranky in the morning. Interestingly, some women do not experience sweats at all, while others sweat both night and day. Some women sweat just at night. No matter which woman you are, sweating is considered to be a severe symptom of perimenopause and menopause because it causes more discomfort and disruption to our daily lives.

These sweating episodes usually come right after a hot flash and begin in your upper body. When sweating is mild, you might just lightly perspire and have a dewy glow to your face. If severe, you will get drenched. I really mean *drenched*. Your whole head will be wet and your hairdo will be absolutely ruined! And if you are sweating at night, you will, at the very least, wake up long enough to toss off your blanket and turn on your fan. If your sweats are really bad, you might even have to change your sheets and get into dry pajamas. I have personally found that wearing a big nightshirt, while not even remotely sexy, makes for a fast and easy nighttime wardrobe change.

The Epic Bedroom Temperature Battle

I often sleep with both the air conditioner and fan on. My husband complains that our bedroom is freezing. I snap back with "Put on a sweater!" And if I awaken in the night in a sweat, I can barely see my husband because the covers are pulled up to his eyeballs.

There is no winning this battle.

There is only compromise.

WHAT CAUSES A HOT FLASH?

Despite the fact that we can put a man on the moon and even get a close-up look at Pluto, we still have no idea what causes a hot flash. What we do know is that some of you appear to have more sensitive thermostats than others, meaning that you feel comfortable only within a small range of temperatures. This range, called a "thermo-neutral zone," is the ideal. If you leave this comfort zone, moving up the temperature scale, you will experience a hot flash. So every time you enter a warm room, engage in exercise, or drink a hot beverage—all activities that raise your core body temperature—you will leave your thermoneutral zone. Subsequently, your body will likely respond with a hot flash.

The signal for this temperature regulation seems to originate in an area of the brain known as the hypothalamus. When your hypothalamus senses that you are too warm, it starts a process to cool you down by dilating blood vessels at the surface of your skin. That is when you experience a hot flash. Odd as it sounds, a hot flash is actually a cooling mechanism. If you need even more cooling down, your brain sends out a signal to add in sweating. Drinking a cold beverage or turning on your air conditioner helps you feel better because it gets you back inside that all-important thermoneutral zone.

Have you ever wondered why some of us have mild, manageable hot flashes without sweats, while others end up soaked like soggy rags twenty times a day? There are indeed some reasons for our differences. Smoking cigarettes and being overweight increases your likelihood of having symptoms. For some unknown reason, black and Hispanic women experience more symptoms than white and Asian women. If you suffered from premenstrual symptoms as a younger woman, you are more likely to complain of hot flashes later on. Interestingly, there is a relationship between our mother's menopause transition and symptom severity and our own. If your mom had an easy time with hot flashes, you probably will too. So take a moment to ask your mom about her experience.

By the way, perimenopause and menopause are not the only

reasons that women can experience hot flashes. Other causes include thyroid disease, infection, cancer, some antidepressants, and certain estrogen-blocking drugs like tamoxifen, which is used to treat breast cancer, and raloxifene, a medication for the treatment of osteoporosis. Night sweats have also been associated with lymphoma and tuberculosis. Your healthcare professional will be able to sort out the origin of your hot flashes by taking a good history and running some blood tests to rule out medical issues like thyroid disease.

Hot Flash Triggers

» Warm rooms
» Hot food
» Spicy food
» Alcohol
» Caffeine
» Stress

HELP IS ON THE WAY!

Are you ready for some wonderful news? It turns out that there are many ways to treat hot flashes and night sweats that can significantly help to reduce your discomfort. I will cover natural choices in chapter 17, "I Want to Feel like a Natural Woman," and pharmacologic options in chapter 16, "Potions, Patches, and Pills, Oh My!"

CHAPTER 3

My Husband Thinks I'm Crazy

Over the next few years, the boardrooms of
America are going to light up with hot flashes.

—GAIL SHEEHY

AT LEAST ONCE A week, I have a new patient tell me that her husband thinks she's lost her mind. My response is always the same. I ask for his name and telephone number and call him right then and there. If I am lucky enough to get him on the line, I introduce myself and explain that his wife is sitting in front of me. Then I say, "Your wife is not crazy. She is just going through perimenopause" or "menopause," whichever the case may be. Husbands are always stunned by my call. I happen to think it is very effective. By the way, you do not have to have a husband or even a partner to hear the words "You're acting crazy!" Your kids, friends, and coworkers will definitely notice if you are moodier. I just don't have time to call everybody.

Are you feeling angry, impatient, anxious, panicky, sad, teary, or just not yourself? It is very common to feel this way during your transition. Changes in mood are experienced by at least 25 percent of women, especially in perimenopause when there are a lot of hormonal ups and downs. Perimenopause is truly marked by hormonal fluctuations. Do you recall my roller-coaster ride analogy in chapter 1, "Girls Are Made of Sugar and Spice and Everything Nice . . . and That Everything Nice Is Estrogen"? Don't worry if you've forgotten that chapter already. I will explain why you are getting so forgetful in chapter 4, "Menofog Rolls In, Focus Rolls Out."

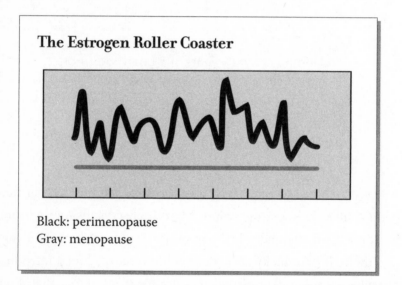

The Estrogen Roller Coaster

Black: perimenopause
Gray: menopause

Menopause is a different story. Hormone levels, particularly estrogen, decline because our ovaries are winding down their duties and heading toward retirement. There are no more hormonal ups and downs, just downs. However, menopause is also marked by many of the same mood changes experienced in perimenopause. Let me give you a typical example of what I hear in my practice.

IT'S NOT JUST IN YOUR HEAD

Not long ago, a forty-five-year-old smart, sophisticated, and generally happy woman walked into my office in tears. I always have a box of tissues on my desk for just such an occasion. She was very upset with herself for overreacting to an issue at work. That led to a downward mood spiral when she returned home and became short-tempered while helping her daughter with homework. My patient admitted to feeling ashamed that she had totally lost her cool. Later on, when no one helped to clear the dinner table, my patient became very angry and practically exploded. That is when she got in her car and drove around for an hour. Talk about road rage. We'd all better steer clear of midlife women drivers who look mad.

But is this behavior considered crazy? Not if you're transitioning through menopause. In fact, many of you can probably tell me your own version of that story. I hope it's a relief to learn that these extremes in mood can often be explained by what is going on between the brain and aging ovaries. Here is how it works:

During our reproductive years, our bodies are designed to ovulate an egg monthly. The brain is responsible for sending signals to the ovary to get this process under way. The ovaries listen to the brain and produce estrogen, progesterone, and testosterone with precise timing. Younger, healthier eggs tend to get chosen for ovulation and potential pregnancy first. That makes sense. Nature wants to put its best foot forward so there is the greatest chance of a successful pregnancy.

What happens later on in our thirties and forties is that we are left with less zesty eggs. That helps explain why women experience issues of infertility and miscarriage as they grow older. Just as it is harder to get these eggs pregnant, it is also harder for them to produce estrogen, progesterone, and testosterone in the right quantity and order. That leads to what happens next.

The brain, and practically every other organ in a woman's body, has receptors for estrogen. When those receptors are filled with estrogen, it's like you are luxuriating in bath oil—you feel so good and relaxed. On the other hand, when those receptors are not filled with estrogen in a reliable and consistent way, the brain becomes unhappy and unsatisfied. Think of your brain as being frustrated and cranky. It begins to send a louder signal to the ovaries to step it up. And therein lies the problem. These aging ovaries cannot do any better. You can no longer depend on them for a regular monthly menstrual cycle. This is perimenopause.

During perimenopause, the ovaries can still make estrogen, but just not reliably and in the right quantity. Sometimes they make too much estrogen. Sometimes they make too little. And other times they get it just right. There is no predictability on a day-to-day or week-to-week basis how this estrogen production facility will perform. So now you can understand why your brain is experiencing a hormonal roller-coaster ride. And hopefully, that helps you understand all of the mood symptoms you have noticed ever since your menstrual cycles started changing.

The good news is that the hormonal swings will stop once you have moved from perimenopause into menopause. The bad news is that because the menopausal ovaries stop producing estrogen altogether, the estrogen receptors in the brain will no longer get their fill. While there will be no more hormonal ups and downs, the lack of estrogen will leave many women more susceptible to feeling "blue," especially if they are experiencing symptoms like hot flashes, night sweats, poor sleep, fatigue, and an overall decreased sense of well-being.

> **Women at a higher risk for mood symptoms often have a history of:**
>
> » PMS
> » Postpartum depression
> » Depression and anxiety earlier on in life

IT'S NOT JUST IN YOUR OVARIES EITHER

So now you know. You are not crazy. Although it is easy to blame hormones for all the moodiness you may be experiencing right now, consider too that there are lots of other reasons that midlife women experience mood changes. What else is going on? This is a time in life when women are often responsible for the care of both their children and their aging parents. How very stressful for everyone involved. I always point out to perimenopausal women that their adolescent daughters are likely on a hormonal roller-coaster ride too. That's why mothers and teenage daughters have difficulties communicating nicely and respectfully with one another. I can still recall being a fifteen-year-old girl and wondering why my forty-five-year-old mother was acting insane. After I grew up and became a specialist in menopausal medicine, I realized that my mother was not crazy but, in fact, perimenopausal!

I have recently begun to experience this mother-daughter rite of passage from the other side. I used to think that when my own daughter got to this stage, I would be able to handle it better than all of you, given my expertise in reproductive endocrinology. Well, ladies, I humbly stand corrected. There is so much sassy sassafras happening in my home, I have begun to think of my once cherubic daughter as Mr. Hyde, the unhinged alter ego of Dr. Jekyll. Wish me luck.

Whether or not you have kids, you probably have aging parents, who are experiencing their own health issues requiring your attention. My father died from complications of Parkinson's disease when I was in my late twenties, and I was not involved in his end of life care. When I was forty years old, my beautiful Momma, Renée, was diagnosed with bone cancer. Although I had just given birth to my daughter weeks before and was exhausted from being up all night breastfeeding and everything else that goes along with new motherhood, I became my mother's patient advocate, escorting her to her medical appointments and sitting by her side during surgery, chemotherapy, bone marrow biopsies, and every single doctor visit thereafter. When I gave birth to my son at forty-one and a half, my mother was in the same hospital getting radiation treatment. I called her right after the birth and told her to wheelchair herself down to me in Labor and Delivery. She was at my side and holding my newborn son within minutes of his birth. Momma died three weeks later.

This was the most stressful time of my life. I want you to know that I have experienced every aspect of the midlife journey. I really do understand what you are going through. I often joke with my husband that we'd better be extra nice to our own children now, so that they will want to take care of us later on.

Midlife is also a time when women face job loss or career changes, financial pressure, difficulties in marriage and other relationships, divorce, widowhood, and health problems. I am sure that you can add to that list of painful life transitions based on your own experience. Patients often tell me that they cannot focus on their own health because they have very busy and stressful lives. I really don't know any women who have it easy. What I do know is that once we hit midlife, the healthy choices we make will resonate all the way to our little old ladyhood.

WHAT WILL HELP?

If you are experiencing distressing changes in mood, it is really important to figure out what's behind it all. Clinical depression and anxiety may be caused by a chemical imbalance in the brain. Alternatively, your feelings of sadness and worry may be attributable to the hormonal changes of perimenopause and menopause.

How does this all get sorted out? What usually happens is that women consult their primary healthcare professional about mood changes and receive a prescription for an antidepressant, anti-anxiety drug, or both. Sometimes a sleep medication is added into the mix too. But if the culprit behind these feelings of sadness, anxiety, anger, and the like are due to the hormonal changes of perimenopause and menopause, this protocol does not usually work out well.

I have a different approach. First, I treat the symptoms of perimenopause and menopause with lifestyle changes like daily exercise and a healthy diet. I also recommend trying de-stressors such as meditation and deep breathing exercises. I may suggest hormonal options, which have a mood-enhancing effect on many women. When menopausal women take estrogen, which I discuss in chapter 16, "Potions, Patches, and Pills, Oh My!," it helps fill up those estrogen receptors in the brain that I told you about earlier. It does not do the job quite like your ovaries did in their prime. Consider it more like a drop in the ocean than a great big wave. However, that drop is enough to flip the switch and positively affect mood.

More often than not, mood symptoms and sleep issues improve significantly with the use of hormone therapy, especially when there are also complaints of hot flashes and night sweats. That is when I get a happy call or e-mail from my own patients letting me know they are feeling much better. In fact, I also become popular with husbands, partners, coworkers, and kids, who definitely notice the improvement. I love those calls and e-mails. Keep them coming. I like to joke that my strategy for getting into heaven someday is by helping out one woman at a time. With *Menopause Confidential,* and the millions of you who will find solutions and relief, I will be in like Flynn!

Sometimes, though, mood symptoms do not improve enough or at all. That is when it's appropriate to explore the use of other medications and psychotherapy for the treatment of depression and anxiety. What if you already take medication for depression, anxiety, or sleep? Well, if you land on my doorstep, I do not discontinue treatment until we have tried and succeeded with my usual approach of lifestyle changes and possibly hormone therapy. Then, in collaboration with your primary healthcare professional, we begin the process of tapering off the mood and sleep aids. Sometimes it works out smoothly. Sometimes it doesn't. That is why I really encourage collaboration to determine the best course of action. When it comes to figuring all this out, it really does take a village.

Signs of Clinical Depression

See your healthcare professional if you experience the following daily symptoms for more than two weeks:

» Depressed mood
» Feelings of hopelessness
» Markedly decreased interest in most activities
» Trouble sleeping or sleeping too much
» Loss or increase in appetite
» Extreme fatigue or loss of energy
» Feelings of worthlessness
» Decreased concentration
» Thoughts of death or suicide

FREE TO BE YOU AND ME

As we end this chapter, I want to leave you with the hope and confidence that you will indeed feel like yourself again. There are many ways to improve mood symptoms during perimenopause and menopause. It takes time and patience to find the right solution. The key is not to give up. It really does start with one step at a time. That is why I am going to shut off my computer and go for a walk in Central Park with my dog, Sadie. That will definitely make me feel better.

Why don't you go for a walk too? All you have to do is slip on your comfortable shoes, put one foot in front of the other, and head out the door. Even though your chores will still be waiting for you when you return, I know that your mood will improve once you have carved out some quality time for your health. Sadie and I will meet you in the park.

CHAPTER 4

Menofog Rolls In, Focus Rolls Out

I must admit I am nervous about getting
Alzheimer's. Once it hits, I might tell
my best joke and never know it.

—JOAN RIVERS

WHAT IS THE NAME of the band that sings your favorite song from
the seventies? You love that song. Or how about those famous
movie stars in that great movie, you know the one with Rob Reiner's
mother at Katz's deli? The answers are hovering on the edge of your
brain. Why won't they roll off your tongue? This is often where husbands and partners come in handy. Between the two of you, the
answers get figured out eventually . . . Fleetwood Mac! Billy Crystal
and Meg Ryan! Thank goodness I remembered, or I would have
driven myself crazy.

You walk into your bedroom, stop, and look around dumb-founded. "What did I come in here to get?" No idea. Maybe if you walk out and come back later, your brain will remember. You have always been so good at focusing. Back in the day, you even read through the fine print in appliance manuals that most of us ignore. Now you are finding it hard to concentrate on reading this paragraph.

Let me reassure you that it is *very* unlikely that you are seeing the first signs of dementia. One of the biggest concerns women have as we get older is whether or not we will end up suffering from Alzheimer's disease, which is the most common type of dementia. In my medical experience, this fear falls right behind that of breast cancer in the overall ranking of what women worry most about as they march through menopause. I think you'll feel better once I clarify some definitions and clear up some myths about our cognitive abilities as we age.

THE AGING BRAIN

Memory, concentration, learning, problem-solving, and reasoning skills all tend to decline as we grow older, and by "older," I mean fifty! And while that expression about growing older and wiser is definitely true, a lot of our wisdom is more likely coming from life experience rather than from any new skills our brain has mastered. It is considered a normal part of aging to have some difficulty remembering certain facts, people, and places. Later on, I will review strategies to keep your brain healthy and sharp.

The menopause transition is a particularly challenging time for women, because this is often when you personally experience more difficulty with *verbal* memory. Verbal memory has to do with recalling words. Part of the explanation for this timing has to do with the fact that the classic symptoms—hot flashes, night sweats, poor sleep, fatigue, and mood changes—can make cognitive ability even worse. However, even women who are not having symptoms will complain of forgetfulness and focus issues. In fact, 60 percent of you, particularly during perimenopause and early menopause when your hormones are still fluctuating, will notice that your brain is not working at its very best. I am happy to report that the further along we get past the menopause transition, the less of a problem this will be for most of us. By the way, this whole constellation of symptoms often gets tossed into one bag called brain fog, or as I like to say, *menofog.*

Menofog Symptoms

» Fogginess
» Forgetfulness
» Lack of focus

Women often joke that their brain fog is a sure sign that dementia is approaching. But, of course, it's not. Dementia refers to a *severe* loss of intellectual ability and is diagnosed when our memory and other brain function duties decline enough to significantly interfere with our independence and the performance of regular daily activities. Dementia is not forgetting someone's name for a few minutes or wondering why you came into a room. It is characterized by not being able to remember how to get home or whether you have eaten. The typical brain fog complaints associated with perimenopause and menopause do not come anywhere close to the severity of those linked to dementia.

Although there are other causes of dementia, Alzheimer's disease is the most common form and usually affects women over the age of sixty-five. But it really is a disease of older women, and the number affected by Alzheimer's makes a great leap once women hit their eighties. Although healthcare professionals can reasonably diagnose Alzheimer's earlier than ever before, the only way to actually confirm the diagnosis is by performing an autopsy, which will show characteristic amyloid plaques and neurofibrillary tangles in the brain.

Risks for Alzheimer's Disease

» Age 65 and older
» Family history
» High blood pressure
» Diabetes
» Abnormal cholesterol
» Stroke
» Repeated head injury

Decrease Your Risk

» Exercise regularly
» Eat a healthy diet
» Maintain a normal weight
» Reduce stress
» Engage in social activities
» Challenge your brain
» Wear your seatbelt and bike helmet

THE MIDLIFE BRAIN

Now let's focus, if we can, on why so many of us complain during the menopause transition of the inability to recall words and concentrate, and why we generally have a harder time learning new things. Part of that is definitely due to the brain aging. The other part is due to the fact that our brain is rich in estrogen receptors that are not getting their fill of the hormone. So it makes perfect sense that when estrogen levels fluctuate in perimenopause and decline in menopause, our brain may not be firing on all pistons. I think of the younger brain as a team of healthy neurons and blood vessels making all kinds of superhighway connections to allow us to function at our highest cognitive capacity. When those neurons and vessels start getting older, and in the absence of a reliable estrogen supply, they cannot possibly make those same swift connections.

The truly exciting news here is that there are many ongoing areas of investigation within the study of menopause and cognition. You and I really don't have time to squander waiting for the results, though, so let's start making some important and scientifically proven lifestyle choices that can help relieve menofog symptoms and protect against dementia now. As it turns out, these very same choices improve total body health and wellness, so we really do get a big bang for our buck.

The best evidence out there for the prevention of cognitive decline points to engaging in regular *aerobic* exercise. Other lifestyle choices that appear to help include maintaining a social network, learning new skills, keeping mentally active, eating a nutritious diet rich in omega-3 fatty acids, not smoking, and reducing the risk for high blood pressure, diabetes, and high cholesterol through regular exercise, healthful eating, and, if necessary, medication.

Supplements of any kind do not appear to help improve brain fog or protect against significant cognitive decline. So save your money.

Once you have read chapter 15, "I Left My Heart in San Francisco," you will notice that what is good for the brain is also good for the heart. But first make sure to bone up on chapter 14, "Sticks and Stones Can Break Your Bones"! You will see clearly that healthier lifestyle choices positively affect you from top to bottom. So for those of you who are either experiencing memory issues or are really worried about Alzheimer's disease, get a move on!

HORMONE THERAPY AND MENOFOG

Spoiler alert. You are going to learn quite a lot about hormone therapy in chapter 16, "Potions, Patches, and Pills, Oh My!" For now, I shall just tease the topic with a question. What role does hormone therapy play in the improvement of brain fog? Well, researchers are still struggling with a definitive answer. Everyone, however, is in agreement that if you are suffering from hot flashes and sweats and choose hormone therapy to improve those symptoms, you will see some collateral benefit to your memory, concentration, focus, and clarity. Women often describe the feeling as having the fog lifted. In fact, I had a patient who was using hormone therapy for her significant night sweats. Within a few months, her head was so much clearer and sharper that she finished a PhD thesis she had started twenty years earlier. That really is a true story.

If you are a younger woman who has undergone a surgical menopause, I should point out that your overall symptom profile will be much more severe. That's because your brain will not have had time to acclimate to a more gradual decline in estrogen levels.

So the recommendation for you in terms of estrogen use for the improvement of cognition is even more strongly supported.

There is also an important concept you should be aware of called the *critical window hypothesis,* which has really gained traction in the medical research community. In a nutshell, it refers to the fact that, as I just noted, when menopausal women use estrogen therapy to treat their hot flashes and night sweats, they also experience improvement of their brain fogginess and verbal memory. But—and this is key—it is essential to get the estrogen supply to the brain early in the menopause transition while those neurons are younger and healthier. Timing appears to be everything. This explains why offering hormone therapy to older women, who are further away from their last menstrual period, is really "too little too late." It may even be harmful: the Women's Health Initiative (WHI), which I will review later, has found that it is in fact a bad idea to offer estrogen for the very first time to women who are more than ten years past their last menstrual period.

There are, however, two very recent clinical trials known as KEEPS and ELITE, which show that younger symptomatic women who use hormone therapy do not increase their risk of dementia. I hope this is reassuring to all of you midlife women who want to try hormone therapy and are afraid because of what you've heard in the news. I will cover the WHI, KEEPS, ELITE, and other landmark studies in chapter 19, "The Top Five Studies That Rocked Women's Health." In general, though, a good guideline to go by is that if you are less than ten years from your last menstrual period, you are still a candidate to try hormone therapy. But don't wait that long. It is much better and safer to initiate therapy right away, when you are having symptoms and are within just a few years of your last period.

Now, here is a mind-boggler. Hormone therapy is only FDA

approved for the treatment of hot flashes, night sweats, and vaginal dryness, not for the treatment of menofog. And despite the fact that selected research suggests that hormone therapy may even help prevent Alzheimer's disease if used early on in the menopause transition, it is not approved for that purpose either. But at least you are now in the know that estrogen really does help with your cognitive complaints and verbal memory. You heard it here first. I hope you remember that.

MEMORIES . . . LIGHT THE CORNERS OF MY MIND

Let's wrap this up with some bottom-line good advice. We should all be proactive when it comes to overall health. The choices we make in our forties and fifties will have a tremendous impact in our eighties. I always tell women that as a physician I need my brain to work at its tip-top capacity and be as sharp as a tack. I am sure you feel the same. So it really is time to get serious about regular daily exercise and a healthy diet. You should consider hormone therapy if you are having hot flashes and night sweats, since you now know there is definitely some benefit to your brain health as well.

By the way, the symptom of brain fog is the very reason I purposefully decided to write a *short* book on menopause. During our menopause transition, most of us will simply not have the cognitive ability to dive deeply into a complicated book with lots of scientific terminology. But take heart. Menofog will not last forever. Our aging brain is constantly adapting, especially when we challenge ourselves. I am giving my fifty-something brain a workout right this minute by writing a book. Julia Child was fifty-one when she first starred in *The French Chef* on TV. I must admit that I love watching the Food Network. I have learned to cook! And . . . Hillary Clinton is running for president of the United States of America at the age of sixty-something. You go, girl!

What new challenge will you take on to improve your brain function? This is not a rhetorical question. I really do expect an answer.

CHAPTER 5

There Is No Rest for the Weary

The best cure for insomnia is to get a lot of sleep.

—W. C. FIELDS

IN MY OPINION, THERE is nothing worse than a bad night's sleep, and nothing better than a good one. When we experience *poor sleep*, which refers to both the amount and quality, we will be tired and cranky the next day. Our ability to focus, concentrate, think clearly, do our work, and take good care of ourselves and everyone else goes to heck in a handbasket. Fatigue and irritability often lead to less healthy food choices and little motivation to exercise. Then comes the inevitable weight gain, which makes most of us even moodier than we already were from lack of sleep. From there, the health consequences just get worse. Did you know that poor sleep increases the risk for heart disease and depression too?

WHAT IS KEEPING YOU UP AT NIGHT?

Sleep issues increase dramatically during perimenopause and menopause and are one of the most common complaints I hear about in my practice. In fact, almost 50 percent of women in their late forties and fifties will experience some degree of sleep disturbance. If it gets really bad, you might even qualify for the dreaded diagnosis of *insomnia*. That means you have difficulty either falling asleep or staying asleep, or you wake up after many hours of sleep not feeling refreshed and restored. As you already know, without enough good sleep, it's much harder to be happy and productive the next day. Despite the fact that sleep issues are twice as common in women, most of the sleep research has been done on men!

THE SLEEP CYCLE TO THE SOUL

Here is how our sleep cycle works. There are four stages, starting with non-rapid eye movement (NREM), which transitions to light sleep, followed by deep sleep, and finally a short period of rapid eye movement (REM) sleep. Then the cycle starts all over again. This cycling occurs several times during the night. We experience more deep sleep in the earlier part of the night and more REM sleep toward the end of the sleep period. The more deep sleep we get, the more rested and restored we feel in the morning. The more REM sleep we get, the better our mood and brain function. It turns out that 80 percent of our sleep is spent in the first three stages, and the remaining 20 percent is devoted to REM.

Unfortunately, midlife women appear to spend more time in light sleep and less time in deep sleep, as compared to younger women. The more time we spend in light sleep, the less refreshed we feel in the morning. And let me introduce yet another sleep disruptive factor that affects us during the menopausal transition— depression, or at the very least, a depressed mood. Poor sleep affects our good mood the next day, and feeling depressed affects our good sleep that night. It's a vicious cycle.

There are plenty of nonmedical reasons causing midlife women to experience problems with sleep, especially nighttime awakening. Difficulties with work, finances, relationships, snoring spouses, children having bad dreams, and aging parents who are not listening to your advice are enough reasons to keep women up at night feeling anxious and depressed. Just getting older is associated with having less sleep overall.

By the way, I would also like to add pets to the list of reasons that contribute to sleep disruption. My dog, Sadie, woke me up several times last night. So it is extremely ironic that in my current sleep-deprived state, I am writing a chapter on sleep disturbances.

WHEN SNORING IS NOT BORING

Of course, there are also some specific medical reasons that cause midlife women to experience sleep disturbances. I would like to give a special shout-out to the women who experience sleep apnea, a condition that involves disruptive pauses in breathing several times during the night and which is specifically associated with loud snoring and daytime sleepiness. You are at particular risk for high blood pressure and sudden cardiac death. So for all of you loud snorers, you really should be evaluated at a sleep center. That also goes for all the true insomniacs out there. Your health is at stake.

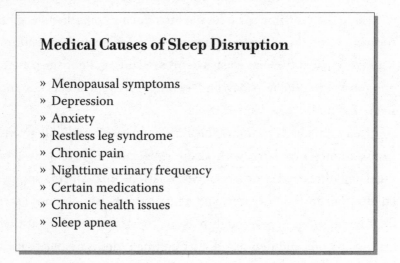

Medical Causes of Sleep Disruption

» Menopausal symptoms
» Depression
» Anxiety
» Restless leg syndrome
» Chronic pain
» Nighttime urinary frequency
» Certain medications
» Chronic health issues
» Sleep apnea

A MYSTERY WORTHY OF SHERLOCK HOLMES

Now here comes a midlife medical mystery. Despite the fact that you and I are both convinced that our hot flashes and night sweats are waking us up, many scientific studies that have sought to prove this cause and effect have not clearly made the connection. It seems so obvious. However, it turns out that not every woman wakes up after a nighttime flash or sweat. Plenty of women sleep right through their symptoms with no problem. There is also evidence that perhaps it's the awakening that happens first, which then triggers the flashing and sweating.

And then there are the very real midlife issues of depression and anxiety, which influence both our menopause symptoms as well as our sleep quality. No matter what comes first, the chicken or the egg, midlife women wake up a lot. Some of us will be drenched or just very hot, and that is the end of our chance at getting a good night's sleep. Others will feel anxious and depressed. And most of us will feel lousy the next day. By the way, I hear from a lot of you that you spend your late-night awake time doing Internet searches looking for solutions to improve sleep, hot flashes, and night sweats!

Of course, many of the symptoms of menopause, like fatigue, moodiness, and brain fog, would certainly improve if only women could get a good night's sleep. Or is it the other way around? Would your sleep improve if your nighttime flashes and sweats subsided? I will answer the question of which came first, the chicken or the egg, in chapter 16, "Potions, Patches, and Pills, Oh My!"

BETTER THAN COUNTING SHEEP

So what solutions are available for midlife women's sleep issues? The nonprescription strategies appear to start with the same life-style recommendations we have already talked about, including a healthy diet, daily exercise, weight maintenance, and not smoking. It turns out that nicotine makes it both harder to fall as well as stay asleep. Additionally, while alcohol makes many of us feel sleepy, it ultimately disrupts our sleep later on. Caffeine from coffee, tea, soda, chocolate, nonprescription pain relievers, allergy and cold medications, and weight-loss drugs will also keep us from getting the sleep we need. I think about that every time my husband orders the chocolate molten cake. I usually indulge in just one bite for this very reason. And I never order a postdinner cappuccino anymore.

In fact, eating a large or heavy meal near bedtime will also make it harder to sleep. I no longer make fun of older people eating dinner at the early bird special hour. I've joined them at the table!

Additional nonprescription sleep strategies include maintaining good sleep habits. That means you have to establish a sleep routine that you stick to every night of the week. You must go to bed and wake up around the same time whenever possible. Your bed and bedding must be comfortable. Keep your bedroom cool, dark, and quiet. Reading in bed is okay, unless you have chosen a scary Stephen King novel. Watching TV in bed is *not* okay. Nor is working on your computer and smartphone. If you must do those activities, sit in the living room until you feel sleepy.

Good Sleep Habits

» Go to bed around the same time each night
» Keep your bedroom cool, dark, and quiet
» Buy a comfortable mattress, bedding, and pillows
» Don't watch TV or use a computer in bed
» Leave your charging smartphone in another room
» Exercise daily and only during the day
» Eat dinner early
» Avoid alcohol and caffeine close to bedtime
» Never, ever smoke cigarettes
» Wear earplugs if you're sensitive to sound
» Stick to your routine, and your sleep will improve!

You can try yoga, acupuncture, and meditation to improve your sleep, although there is not enough good research on whether these activities make any difference. The same is true for botanical supplements and over-the-counter melatonin. My feeling about these strategies is that if you want to try something that your best friend swears by, go ahead. However, if it does not help you after three months, it's time to move along.

In addition to my dog and kids, I have to include my husband on the list of issues that keep me from my beauty rest. Practically every night, he winds up falling asleep in his home office with both the TV blaring and the computer beaming. Then I have to get out of bed to turn off all the electronics. I should probably also admit that I am guilty of the TV-in-bed transgression. Besides watching the cooking shows, I also indulge in *The Real Housewives of Beverly Hills, New Jersey,* and, of course, *New York City.* But I always turn off the tube by 10:00 PM That's when I tackle the *New York Times,* which really knocks me right out.

PRESCRIPTION STRENGTH

Finally, let's talk about prescription solutions for midlife women who are experiencing sleep disturbances or insomnia. Your healthcare professional can offer short-acting sleeping pills like Ambien that work well. But there is always a concern that you may also experience sleepiness the next day, or develop a tolerance to their initial effects or, worst of all, a dependence on them. I do think that short-acting sleeping pills are helpful for women when the cause of the sleep disturbance is stress-related. If you cannot sleep because you are dealing with illness, divorce, job loss, or death of a loved one, consider talking to your healthcare professional about getting a prescription. Sleeping pills can also help you slumber on a long, overnight plane ride so you feel refreshed when you arrive at that faraway place you have always dreamed about. For these short-term problems, medication can provide real benefits.

HORMONES TO THE RESCUE!

Here is how hormone therapy shakes out with regard to improving sleep. There are estrogen receptors located in specific areas of the brain that are responsible for regulating body temperature, mood, and sleep. So if you are having hot flashes, night sweats, and mood issues, then hormone therapy will certainly improve those symptoms and, therefore, help you sleep better. That is especially true when using an oral estrogen and a natural progesterone tablet. However, I also see improvement when women take non-oral estrogen, which you will read about in chapter 16, "Potions, Patches, and Pills, Oh My!" By the way, the progesterone tablet is taken at bedtime *because* it can cause drowsiness. What a delightful side effect to have when you are experiencing sleep issues!

Even if you are not flashing and sweating at night, hormone therapy still appears to benefit sleep especially by reducing the number of times you wake up. The bottom line is that midlife women report that they generally feel more rested after they start hormone therapy. However, hormone therapy should not be used for the sole purpose of improving sleep. It really is only FDA-approved for the treatment of hot flashes, night sweats, and vaginal dryness, a topic that I will cover in the next chapter, "The Vagina Is like Las Vegas, *Baby!*"

MY QUEENDOM FOR A GOOD NIGHT'S SLEEP

I would like to end this chapter on an empathetic note. Most of us would like to make the necessary lifestyle changes on our journey to midlife health and wellness. Yet fatigue and daytime sleepiness, along with a depressed mood, can make this practically impossible. For instance, it really would be great to lose ten pounds. But the reality is that eating healthier and exercising more is hard to do when you feel so tired and miserable. My advice to my own patients is to start with one change for the better. We can all do that. What change are you going to make today? Feel free to e-mail me your answer!

CHAPTER 6

The Vagina Is Like Las Vegas, *Baby*!

> I was worried about vaginas. I was worried
> about what we think about vaginas, and even
> more worried that we don't think about them.
>
> —EVE ENSLER

WHAT GOES IN THE vagina stays in the vagina! Have I got your attention? A few years ago, I made that statement on *The Dr. Oz Show* while talking about vaginal health during perimenopause and menopause. It definitely made the audience sit up and listen closely. This is my favorite way to introduce a very important topic that causes so many of you great embarrassment. I will get to exactly why the vagina is like Las Vegas momentarily.

THE CHANGING VAGINA

Here is the inconvenient truth. All of us will begin to experience vulvar and vaginal changes, collectively referred to as atrophy, once we begin our menopause transition. These changes are caused by a decrease in estrogen levels, which leads to thinning, dryness, decreased elasticity, and even inflammation of vulvar and vaginal tissues. I like to think of the vulva and vagina as becoming more dainty and delicate. Because of that, at least 50 percent of us will experience some degree of burning, irritation, and itchiness within a few years of our last menstrual period. And for those of you who are sexually active, sex will very likely be painful. As I always say to my patients, no woman in the world will be interested in sex if it hurts.

When Senator Bob Dole was on a television commercial years ago to discuss erectile dysfunction and Viagra, he helped pave the way for midlife men to have active sex lives. All of a sudden, men had a solution to their problem. They were ready to go! But their partners, women in perimenopause and menopause, were not. In fact, back in that Dark Age, midlife women were lagging far behind in terms of addressing their own sexual health.

Dare I say that many of you are still in the dark, so let me turn on a light. For those who are interested, there is something that can and should be done to improve your sex life. It all starts with maintaining both vulvar and vaginal health. And it doesn't matter to me if you aren't sexually active. Every woman is entitled to a healthy vagina, whether she is using it or not! That sounds like it could be the beginning of a global initiative. Who will join me?

AN ANATOMY LESSON

The vulva is everything you can see on the outside of your vagina, which is, of course, located inside and therefore can really be visualized only with the help of that cold, metal tool your gynecologist uses, called a speculum. Both the vulva and vagina are estrogen dependent, and they suffer just as much as the rest of you once you are no longer making your own estrogen. Also, there is an entire community of helpful bacteria and other microorganisms that live in the vagina and make it a very hospitable environment that protects us from infections. The whole bacterial and pH balance changes during the menopause transition and that, too, contributes to the symptoms of dryness, burning, irritation, itchiness, discharge, and pain with penetration. For some of you, your annual GYN exam will become a dreaded experience, because the insertion of a speculum will cause more discomfort than you have ever known.

I get very upset when I hear that some healthcare professionals do not devote the time necessary to explain the importance of maintaining vulvar and vaginal health. I understand why it happens, though. Many people find that this is not an easy topic to bring up and discuss openly. So it's really up to you to ask your healthcare professional about it. Consider this a call to arms . . . or more specifically, vaginas!

By the way, there are many other reasons women experience vulvar and vaginal discomfort and symptoms that have nothing to do with perimenopause and menopause. The laundry list of instigators include infections from yeast or bacteria; sexually transmitted diseases like herpes, genital warts, or trichomoniasis; a skin condition known as lichen sclerosis; a chronic pain condition called vulvodynia; vulvar and vaginal cancer; pelvic radiation for certain cancers; and allergic reactions to soap, detergent, body cream, condoms, feminine hygiene products, and much more. I have just given you yet another great reason why you really do need to show up for your annual GYN visit!

BE GOOD TO YOUR BLADDER

Let me introduce you to a relatively new term, *genitourinary syndrome of menopause*. Not only does it refer to the issues we have been discussing about vulvar and vaginal atrophy, but it also includes problems related to the bladder and urethra. The bladder and urethra sit right on top of the vagina and are also dependent on estrogen for health and normal functioning. In the absence of estrogen, you may start experiencing frequent bladder infections or just symptoms of burning and urgency with urination. So if you don't take good care of your vagina, your bladder will suffer too. I will discuss this syndrome more thoroughly in chapter 8, "To Pee or Not to Pee."

YOUR VAGINA HOMEWORK ASSIGNMENT

There are many effective nonmedical treatments to help prevent and treat vulvar and vaginal atrophy after menopause. I always start by recommending to my patients what I call their "weekly homework assignment." This essentially means masturbation, with or without a vibrator. Although this recommendation may surprise some of you, it is the most inexpensive and natural way to achieve the health goal, because it increases blood flow to the genital tissues.

What if you have no libido, are tired, or are just too busy to bother? I offer you the motivation of improved vulvar, vaginal, and bladder health. Just like we have to engage in aerobic exercise for our hearts and strength training for our bones, we also have to do something to help out our pelvic area. It's the very least we can all do to prevent a major quality-of-life issue down the menopause road. And this homework assignment is for every woman, whether you are sexually active or not. Do not get frustrated if you are having difficulty achieving orgasm. The goal is health, so just do the best you can. This homework is supposed to be fun! Now if you do happen to have an active sex life, you are likely already achieving health and wellness of your private bits, so no need to go for extra credit . . . unless you want to!

There are natural vaginal moisturizers, like olive or vitamin E oil, which you rub directly onto the vulva and vagina, to improve dryness. No need to buy expensive extra-virgin olive oil for this purpose—the less expensive stuff works just fine. Many of you ask about whether you can use coconut, almond, vegetable oil, or anything on the shelf that says "oil." The safest answer is "No." It is better to treat your dry vulva and vagina with products that have actually been studied.

By the way, vaginal moisturizers are different from lubricants. Moisturizers need to be used several times a week to get long-term relief from dryness. They work by holding water on to the surface of vaginal cells. Moisturizers are not applied right before sex. Vaginal lubricants, on the other hand, are used for immediate and temporary relief of the discomfort associated with the insertion of a penis or vibrator during sex. They minimize friction and irritation around the clitoris, labia, and vaginal entrance and come in the form of a gel or liquid. Slather some on your partner's private parts too for maximum slipperiness.

You can find many over-the-counter choices for both moisturizers, like Replens and Luvena, and lubricants, like K-Y Jelly and Astroglide, at your local pharmacy. Now that you know the difference between the two, just make sure to check the label so that you don't buy one when you really want the other.

WHY IS THE VAGINA LIKE LAS VEGAS?

Here is the moment you have all been waiting for, the secret meaning behind my chapter title revealed! It is my way of helping you understand how *local* vaginal estrogen is different from *systemic* estrogen. When using a local estrogen preparation directly on the vulva and vagina to treat menopause-related atrophy and symptoms, you are not putting your breasts at risk for cancer, something that many of you have heard is associated with all hormone therapy. This is a very important concept to grasp, and a very big reason women are not using estrogen to tend to their vaginas. The *local* estrogen preparation is not significantly absorbed into the bloodstream. That means that the estrogen does not leave the vagina and travel elsewhere in the body, like to the breast. So women can use local vaginal estrogen to treat their dry vaginas without worrying about increasing their breast cancer risk. In fact, breast cancer survivors can safely use local vaginal estrogen to prevent and treat their symptoms of vaginal dryness and painful intercourse. And believe me, they do!

There are several FDA-approved local estrogen preparations available for the treatment of menopause-related vulvar and vaginal atrophy, and I will discuss them in detail in chapter 16, "Potions, Patches, and Pills, Oh My!" Local estrogen restores blood flow, improves tissue elasticity and vaginal pH, and plumps up the cells so they can resume their ability to lubricate once again, just like in the good old days. That is the key difference between estrogen and nonhormonal treatments, which do not restore the physiologic health of the vulvar and vaginal tissues. Even though the FDA currently mandates that the informational package insert for local vaginal estrogen preparations carry the same warnings as the systemic estrogens (such as the risk of breast cancer), you are now in-the-know and actually know more on this topic than most healthcare professionals.

So viva Las Vegas! When it comes to local estrogen use, what goes in the vagina really does stay in the vagina!

LET'S TALK ABOUT SEX

The discussion of normal sexual function in perimenopause and menopause starts with vulvar and vaginal health. However, it does not end there. At least 50 percent of you will also complain of decreased libido, even after vaginal health is restored and intercourse is comfortable. Libido turns out to be a very complicated topic with many factors involved. Our brain is a critical part of our normal sexual function, and without estrogen *and* testosterone filling up our brain receptors, we cannot possibly have the same sexual interest we once did.

As you might remember from our earlier discussion about hormones, women make plenty of testosterone, and it plays a big role in our sex drive. We have twice as much testosterone in our twenties as we do in our sixties. So not only does our libido drop, but achieving orgasm also takes longer—if we can even get there at all. If we do, it probably will not feel as intense as it once did. However, let me assure you that having a reduced libido is normal for most of us as we age. That does not mean we cannot have a satisfying sex life, if we want one. I will talk more about the hormonal options that improve sexual function in chapter 16, "Potions, Patches, and Pills, Oh My!"

By the way, it's ironic that I am writing this chapter the very same week that a new drug, flibanserin, has been approved for pre-menopausal women who suffer from hypoactive sexual desire disorder (HSDD). To get that diagnosis, you have to have had a normal interest in sex at one time and feel distress that you do not have desire now. You cannot be diagnosed with HSDD if your reason for low libido is not having a partner, not liking your partner, or having a partner with his or her own sexual function issues. Likewise if you are experiencing an illness; taking certain medications like anti-depressants that are known to reduce libido; dealing with meno-pause symptoms, weight gain, depression, anxiety, or insomnia; or simply just being an exhausted working woman who is busy raising kids and caring for elderly parents and therefore too pooped to pop. So before you go sprinting to your healthcare professional's office for a prescription, you should know that they must be specially cer-tified before they can offer this drug, *and* you must answer a ques-tionnaire to determine if you really have HSDD and are a candidate.

DID YOU KNOW?

Here is a fun fact. When sex is good, it adds 15 to 20 percent addi-tional value to a relationship. But when sex is bad or nonexistent, it tosses about 50 to 70 percent of the positive value right out the win-dow. So if you are interested in having a healthy and satisfying sex life, it is time to speak openly and honestly about your own physical changes, especially with your partner. I will steer you in the right direction in chapter 20, "Every Man Needs a Gynecologist."

Let's end this chapter with another homework assignment. Ladies, do not forsake your vaginas any longer! Make it *your* responsibility to start the conversation about your own sexual health and wellness today.

Homework is due in one month!

CHAPTER 7

What's the Skinny on Weight Gain?

Middle age is when your age starts
to show around your middle.

—BOB HOPE

IF I HAD A nickel for every time I heard "I have tried everything, and I simply cannot lose weight!" I would have a lot of nickels. Believe me, if I sent you to the *Survivor* island with a box of raisins, you would lose those extra pounds. All kidding aside, I really do know the secret to weight loss, because I understand the reasons behind weight gain. And once you do too, you will be able to make the necessary changes toward your own health and wellness. And just for the record, our goal at midlife should be to maximize health. So instead of focusing on *weight loss*, repackage your goal as *health gain*. That sounds loftier.

THE REASONS BEHIND OUR BIGGER BEHIND

The menopause transition is a time when women complain vociferously about gaining weight. I can hear you now. Gone are the days when we can skip just one meal and fit comfortably into our jeans. No longer can we take an exercise class and expect to topple our muffin tops. All of a sudden, we wake up to find that our bellies have gotten bigger and our zippers have gotten tougher to close. Inevitably, we are driven to purchase too many pairs of black pants and skirts from Chico's. And don't forget about Spanx, which is really just a fancy name for a girdle. Midlife is indeed associated with both a redistribution of fat—it lands smack dab in our middle—as well as a reduction in lean body mass. This midlife malady has a name. Let me introduce you to your menopot.

It is more than fair to say that the symptoms we experience during our transition, like hot flashes, night sweats, and poor sleep, do indeed contribute to our overall fatigue. And tired women are less inclined to take a SoulCycle class or turn down a delicious Boston cream donut. In fact, sleep deprivation has been scientifically linked to weight gain. Please review chapter 5, "There Is No Rest for the Weary," for tips on getting a good seven hours of restorative rest.

Furthermore, as we age, our metabolism begins to slow down, making it harder to burn off calories. And unfortunately, even though we need fewer calories, we still want to eat, drink, and party like it was 1999. Finally, our muscle mass decreases, and thus our ability to burn calories is less efficient. You will learn more about that in chapter 18, "Do I Really Have to Lift Weights Too?"

So now you know the real culprit behind weight gain at midlife. It is your aging body and the fact that you are not making the necessary lifestyle changes required to accommodate your change of life. I know you really wanted to hear that weight gain is the fault of menopause. If only it were that simple!

YOU CAN'T ALWAYS EAT (AND DRINK) WHAT YOU WANT!

Every five years, the United States Departments of Agriculture (USDA) and Health and Human Services (HHS) release new and improved "Dietary Guidelines for Americans" to facilitate healthier *eating patterns* based on the latest scientific evidence. As it turns out, our *pattern of eating* is much more important in the overall health scheme of things than the occasional guilty food indulgence. Fifty-two percent of the vegetables that Americans eat are tomatoes and potatoes, mostly in the form of French fries, potato chips, ketchup, and tomato sauce on pizza. And we eat only half of the daily recommended allowance of fruits and vegetables. If we develop healthy eating patterns *early in life*, that will translate into maintaining a healthy weight and preventing chronic diseases later on.

As an aside, I think I speak for a generation of women who grew up in the late 1960s and 1970s when I say that Swanson frozen fried-chicken dinners, SpaghettiOs, and an assortment of Yodels, Devil Dogs, and Twinkies comprise some of the greatest culinary memories of our childhood. In our defense, the U.S. dietary guidelines did not get issued until the 1980s, so we really can't feel too badly about enjoying all those Ring Dings. However, the processed-food party has long been over. And midlife is the perfect time to get serious about what foods we choose to put into our mouths.

A HEALTHY EATING PATTERN

When women tell me that they are going to consult with a nutritionist to figure out what to eat, I often respond that making healthy food choices really just comes down to common sense. This is not rocket science, so let's not make it any harder than it has to be. And if you are lactose intolerant, vegan, avoiding gluten, or just hate clams, there are still plenty of options for you.

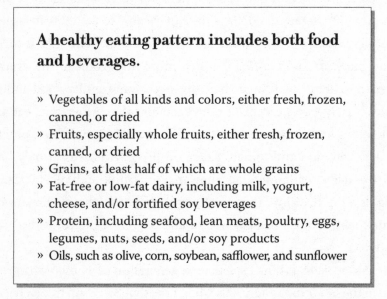

A healthy eating pattern includes both food and beverages.

» Vegetables of all kinds and colors, either fresh, frozen, canned, or dried
» Fruits, especially whole fruits, either fresh, frozen, canned, or dried
» Grains, at least half of which are whole grains
» Fat-free or low-fat dairy, including milk, yogurt, cheese, and/or fortified soy beverages
» Protein, including seafood, lean meats, poultry, eggs, legumes, nuts, seeds, and/or soy products
» Oils, such as olive, corn, soybean, safflower, and sunflower

The big controversy regarding these updated guidelines is that there is no formal recommendation regarding eating *less* red, processed meat and processed poultry to reduce our risk of heart disease and cancer. So I will mention it to you now. We really should eat less of those foods, as you will learn in chapter 15, "I Left My Heart in San Francisco."

I suppose I must address your concerns about carbohydrates. They seem to have gotten a very bad reputation over the past few years. The most popular ones include white bread, potatoes, white rice, pasta, cereal, and soft drinks. However, despite all the fuss, they are not really so terrible after all. An extensive review of the scientific literature has not shown a link between a diet high in carbohydrates and heart disease. Carbohydrates do, however, boost your blood sugar levels and may slightly increase your risk for diabetes. So let's enjoy all of our carbohydrate choices in *moderation.* When you next eat a plate of spaghetti Bolognese, perhaps with a nice glass of Merlot, skip the bread and butter. And the guilt.

> **Added sugar increases the risk of obesity, heart disease, diabetes, and cancer.**

A healthy eating pattern also *limits* saturated and trans fats, added sugars, and salt. Please pay attention to the concept of *added* sugar. Natural sugar in dairy products and fruits are okay. But there are added sugars lurking all around you. Beware of salad dressing, ketchup, and barbecue sauce. Alcohol is full of sugar too.

The specific guidelines for saturated fats, sugars, and salt from "Dietary Guidelines for Americans" are included below. You may need to get out your calculator.

> » Consume <10% of calories/day from added sugars
> » Consume <10% of calories/day from saturated fats
> » Consume <2,300 mg/day of sodium
> » Alcohol should be avoided or consumed in moderation (≤1 drink/day)

If you do not see your favorite foods listed in any of the rec-ommendations above, it's because they did not make the cut for the healthy eating pattern team. That doesn't mean you can't enjoy cake and cookies occasionally. Sadly, I have never seen my all-time favorite food, the barbecue potato chip, on any recommended list anywhere, ever.

A BIG FAT CONTROVERSY

We have all been taught for decades that saturated fat found in meat, butter, and cheese causes heart disease. The proposed mechanism for this association has been the fact that saturated fats increase bad LDL cholesterol. However, a recent analysis of the best scientific evidence to date did not show that people who ate higher levels of saturated fat had more heart disease than those who ate less. To explain this discrepancy, researchers suggest that while saturated fats do indeed raise LDL cholesterol, the elevation occurs in a nicer LDL subtype, described as being big and fluffy, which does not clog up our arteries. Additionally, saturated fats increase good HDL cholesterol.

So what are we to make of this counterintuitive fatty conun-drum? The latest news is not an invitation to eat a high-fat diet. Remember, you are what you eat. So if you eat more fat, you will get fatter. However, we can all take some comfort in the fact that when we indulge in our favorite comfort foods, which are inevitably higher in fat content, we can feel less consumed with guilt about causing a heart attack. Everything in moderation appears to be the best approach to nutritional health, unless one is talking about fruits and vegetables. There are no restrictions on kumquats and kale.

> **Coffee is now included in a healthy eating pattern.**

SHOULD WE ALL MOVE TO THE MEDITERRANEAN?

That will not be necessary, but a nice trip to Greece and a good meal sounds divine. In the meantime, we should eat as if we live there, because a typical Mediterranean diet, which includes more fish, extra-virgin olive oil, vegetables, fruits, legumes, herbs and spices, high-fiber whole grains, nuts, and avocado has definitely been linked to reduced heart attacks and strokes.

THE SECRET TO WEIGHT LOSS

Weight loss comes down to a simple math equation. No calculators are necessary. Think of it as a debit and credit at the calorie bank. In general, we have to eat less. And we also have to eat more. By that, I mean more of the foods that are nutrient rich and healthy. You know which foods I am talking about, since I listed them in the tables above. I have personally incorporated crunchy baby carrots and almonds into my daily diet. Whenever I feel snacky, I reach for my supply. I have also taken quite a liking to Bolthouse Farms 100% carrot juice. The label says that this juice is made from 39¾ carrots. That information alone makes me laugh. I feel healthier and happier with every gulp.

Now here comes a big secret. You can lose weight, even if you never, ever exercise again. But that would be a terrible idea, since physical activity is a critical component to overall health and wellness.

But when it comes to weight loss, the fact of the matter is that exercise will contribute only when we engage in the right *daily* amount.

According to the American Heart Association, women have to exercise for *sixty minutes every single day, seven days a week,* to enjoy the weight-loss benefits. That explains why you are not losing weight despite the fact that you are at the gym three times a week. It turns out not to be enough when it comes to losing weight. I often joke that the only people who have that kind of time are the exercise instructors. The rest of us have to go to work, schlep children hither and thither, go grocery shopping, and then cook dinner.

I use these weight-loss exercise guidelines, however, to motivate my own patients. There is always room for improvement. It may seem like no big deal when a woman gains only one pound at her annual visit. However, this one pound per year turns into those extra ten pounds you are complaining about. And by "you," I also mean me.

THE OPRAH EFFECT

Long before Oprah started touting the benefits of Weight Watchers on TV, I was encouraging my patients to try it. Remember, I have a front-row seat to your weight changes over time. Although many women lose weight on any of those diet plans you hear and read about, the only women who seem to be able to maintain the weight loss are the Weight Watchers. I think it's because you don't have to buy special shakes or premade foods, which never work out when you want to eat at a restaurant. Instead, the Weight Watchers are taught how to eat healthily, no matter what food situation they find themselves in.

I wish I could say that you heard this secret here first. But since Oprah got to you before I could, I would just like to add that Oprah agrees with me.

As an aside, my friend once told me about the only diet that ever worked for her. She calls it the PUSH diet, which means she pushes food away. I am still giggling at the simplicity of this concept. I have tried it, by the way. It definitely works.

MY FIFTIETH BIRTHDAY PARTY MENU

When I turned fifty, I threw myself a disco dance party in the East Village neighborhood where I grew up. I personally chose all my favorite songs and even put them in the precise order that I wanted them to play. My invitation clearly instructed my guests to wear their dancing shoes. I still listen to my awesome playlist when I am walking briskly on my treadmill, as you will learn in chapter 18, "Do I Really Have to Lift Weights Too?"

Despite everything I know about healthy nutrition, when it came time to choose the food I would serve at my party, I picked all the favorites from my youth, a veritable who's who of saturated fat, sugar, and salt. There were buckets of Kentucky Fried Chicken; pans of pierogi, sautéed in buttery onions; and platters of sushi over that delectable sweetened white rice with plenty of salty soy sauce. Yum, yum, yum. For dessert, I served Italian cannoli and pignoli cookies from the venerable Veniero's, and the world-famous prune hamantaschen from Moishe's, both childhood haunts. Lest you think I ignored the health of my guests completely, there was also a very delicious tray of asparagus and a gorgeous mushroom and carrot medley.

I do not feel guilty at all about eating those comfort foods once in a while. For most days of the year, I really do eat healthily. So when I indulge in a pastrami sandwich on rye with Russian dressing and a pickle on the side from the famous 2nd Ave Deli in New York City, I make sure to really enjoy it. It may be years before I get to eat another one.

In the meantime, I am making lots of little dietary changes. A patient once showed me an app that tallies up calories. I typed in my favorite Bombay Sapphire gin martini with *three* olives. I was amazed to learn how many additional calories the three olives added. I now enjoy a martini with just a lemon twist!

Calories Add Up!

Drink	Amount	Calories
Soda	8 oz.	150
Beer	12 oz.	150
Wine	5 oz.	120
Gin	1.5 oz.	97
Scotch	1 oz.	64
Water	A lot!	0

THE VEGGIE WRAP-UP

Now you know everything there is to know about healthy eating, so it's time to start making the changes that will allow you to achieve the ultimate midlife goal of good health and wellness. Remember at the end of *The Wizard of Oz*, when Glinda, the Good Witch, tells Dorothy that the power to go home was always within her? All Dorothy had to do was click her ruby red slippers and believe that she could do it. Well, the same is true for you regarding weight loss and health gain. All you have to do is believe in yourself, and just get the hard work done. No fancy shoes necessary.

By the way, my husband eats an apple a day. That is supposed to keep the doctor away. Do you think my husband is sending me a secret message?

CHAPTER 8

To Pee or Not to Pee

Did you know . . . line dancing was started
by women waiting to use the bathroom.

—ANONYMOUS

LET'S GET SOMETHING CLEARED up right away. Urinary incontinence is not a normal part of aging. I am always dismayed when women tell me that they have completely changed their lifestyle to accommodate their bladders. Do you have to tinkle before you leave your home and then again immediately upon arrival at your destination? Are you constantly scoping out where all the restrooms are at the mall, movie theatre, and nearest restaurant? Have you resorted to wearing a sanitary napkin every day? Many women answer "Yes" to all of the above. And my response to that is "No!" Your life should not revolve around the nearest bathroom.

Urinary incontinence is a major quality-of-life issue. And despite the fact that 50 percent of us will experience leakage at some point, we cannot blame menopause and declining estrogen levels. We can, however, implicate the following factors that do increase our risk of incontinence, including advancing age, diabetes, obesity, hysterectomy, and childbirth. For some of us, age brings along frailty, a slower gait, and therefore difficulty walking to the bathroom quickly enough. The other listed risk factors can lead to pelvic organ prolapse, meaning your uterus, bladder, vagina, and rectum lose their support and start sagging or even falling out of your body.

I will never forget a medical mission I joined in the jungles of Guatemala, where the average patient had given birth to five children. I have never seen such terrible uterine prolapse, where a woman's uterus and bladder were practically hanging down to her knees. I am not exaggerating.

Constipation and the subsequent straining can contribute to prolapse too, so eat your daily fiber. Coughing, by the way, will increase your risk of incontinence. Do I need to give all of the cigarette smokers out there any more reasons to quit?

BLADDER MATTERS

There are basically two types of incontinence, *stress* and *urge*. Stress incontinence will cause you to leak urine when you laugh, sneeze, cough, or jump up and down in exercise class. This annoying condition is the result of having weak pelvic floor muscles, the muscles that support your bladder, urethra, and uterus. When pressure in your belly increases from, say, laughing at a funny joke, it pushes down on your sagging bladder, causing small amounts of urine to leak out. You know that old saying, "I laughed so hard, I peed in my pants." Well, it may capture the experience succinctly, but stress incontinence is no laughing matter.

Urge incontinence develops for a different reason. All of a sudden you will feel the urge to urinate, and large amounts of urine will soak through your panties as a result of an overactive muscle in your bladder that contracts for no apparent reason. If you are very unlucky, you can have a combination of both stress *and* urge incontinence. And with that kind of luck, I would encourage you to stay away from gambling.

There is another condition called overactive bladder syndrome (OAB), which can sometimes look like urge incontinence, although you may very well just have the urge symptoms and not the incontinence. If you have OAB, you will probably have urinary frequency during the day *as well as* during the night. Here is a good rule of thumb: it's considered normal to awaken from sleep just once for tinkling purposes. If you are awakening more than that, it is called *nocturia*, which means waking up frequently at night to tinkle. And that is not normal. I would also like to point out that women with OAB tend to avoid sexual intimacy because of the fear of leaking urine. And that is just a shame.

Even though so many of you will experience urinary incontinence of one kind or another, only half of you are likely to bring up the topic at your annual visit. I think that may be because you are either embarrassed or perhaps think that incontinence is an acceptable part of aging. I always say to my patients, "I will not accept that you are incontinent!" And then we come up with a plan of action. Most of you probably don't realize that there are effective strategies and treatment options that can either cure incontinence or at least significantly improve the symptoms. So let's review them.

WIPING OUT INCONTINENCE

I would like to be the first one to admit that not every gynecologist is an expert in bladder health. I often have to turn to colleagues in urogynecology and urology for help with my own patients. However, there are some simple maneuvers that can and should be done before seeking a specialist. Since weak pelvic floor muscles cause stress incontinence, I thought it might be a good idea to start with a master class in Kegel exercises.

Thank You, Dr. Kegel!

We owe a great debt of gratitude to Dr. Arnold Kegel, an American gynecologist who observed that childbirth weakened the pelvic floor muscles, leading to bladder leakage.

His groundbreaking research in the 1940s demonstrated that exercises could indeed help pelvic floor muscles recover their strength, even after years of disuse, and thereby improve urinary incontinence.

I know that many of you have heard about Kegels. I also know that most of you are not doing them! Here is a good way to look at it. If you want to have great biceps and firm triceps, you have to do the corresponding arm exercises. The only way to get those toned arms is to do the work. The same is true for your pelvic floor musculature. If you want to maintain bladder support, you have to do the Kegels. This involves squeezing the muscles that control the flow of urine, then holding that squeeze for three full seconds . . . 1-one thousand, 2-one thousand, 3-one thousand. How about doing a few squeezes on your morning commute, during that long conference call, or while driving the kids to after-school activities? I am doing my Kegel exercises right now just to prove that we can all do them wherever we are and whenever we want! The secret is out.

Do Your Kegels Daily

» Squeeze the muscles that control urine flow
» Hold for 3 full seconds
» Release the squeeze
» Repeat in sets of 10 for at least 30 per day
» Enjoy laughing again without worry!

STOP THE STRESS

Here is another strategy that helps with stress incontinence. I love pessaries, which hold the bladder and urethra in their proper position. They look like small donut rings and are made out of latex or silicone. You insert one into your vagina and tuck it behind your pubic bone, just as you would insert a diaphragm (for those of you old enough to remember that form of birth control). Pessaries are a great option if you feel comfortable with vaginal insertion. With a little practice, you can easily remove them for intercourse or cleaning. And you will never have to worry about leakage during Zumba class again!

More strategies to reduce stress incontinence include limiting fluid intake when you know you will have trouble getting to a bathroom; tinkling at regular times, even if you do not have the urge; maintaining a normal weight; and, as I mentioned earlier, quitting cigarette smoking so you can reduce coughing. If these self-help strategies are not enough, consult a trained physical therapist, who can teach you pelvic floor biofeedback. The therapist uses sensors to gather information about the way you are using—or not using—your pelvic floor muscles, then helps you learn how to gain control. If you are still experiencing stress incontinence after all of these maneuvers, it is time to see a urogynecologist or urologist to discuss your surgical options.

END THE URGE

You should also turn to a specialist if you think you are experiencing urge incontinence. This is a diagnosis that really should be confirmed through urodynamic testing, which a urogynecologist or urologist can provide. The good news is that urge incontinence usually responds quickly to prescription medications. Avoiding anything that can irritate your bladder, like caffeine, alcohol, nicotine, acidic fruits and vegetables, and spicy foods may help too.

Since 50 percent of women will experience overactive bladder symptoms at some point, we should all consider adopting some helpful strategies like reducing fluid intake right before bedtime, avoiding the bladder irritants noted above, doing our favorite Kegel exercises, and, if necessary, taking a prescription medication to reduce the urge to go, go, go.

INFECTION PREVENTION

As previously mentioned in chapter 6, "The Vagina Is like Las Vegas, *Baby!*," there is a condition called the genitourinary syndrome of menopause that involves changes to the vulva and vagina as well as the bladder and urethra due to declining estrogen levels. Here is where menopause *can* be associated with pee-related problems. Without estrogen, women are more at risk for bladder infections, which can lead to both incontinence and kidney infections. This is *very* important, because kidney infections can kill you. I hope that got your attention. By the way, it's a good bet that you have a bladder infection if you have pain and burning with urination and feel the urge to empty your bladder frequently. Bladder infections are treated with a short course of antibiotics. If possible, it is always better to get a urine culture before you start treatment.

Reduce Your Risk of Infections

» Tinkle before and after sex.
» Tinkle before and after travel.
» Wipe from front to back after urination or a bowel movement.
» Avoid douches, sprays, and other feminine "deodorant" products.
» Wear breathable fabrics to avoid trapping moisture, which encourages bacterial growth.
» Stop wearing tight jeans that cause irritation, lock in moisture, are uncomfortable, and don't even look good anymore!

Now here comes another secret. Drinking cranberry juice or taking cranberry tablets will probably not help prevent or treat a bladder infection. And remember that juice is very high in sugar and calories!

So my final answer to the question "To pee or not to pee" is . . . not to pee . . . unless you want to!

CHAPTER 9

Who Is That Wrinkly Old Woman in the Mirror?

Wrinkles should merely indicate
where smiles have been.

—MARK TWAIN

MY PATIENTS OFTEN ASK me for the secret to my youthful looking skin. My answer is always the same. First, you have to pick your mother correctly, which I did. In other words, I inherited excellent skin genes. Then I stayed out of the sun for many years, because I was holed up in a darkened cubby of the library, studying to become a doctor. Of course, I realize that this formula cannot be applied to everyone. However, just like you, I am also experiencing midlife changes to my skin that have not put a smile on my face. By the way,

I want it on record that I am very proud of my smile lines. I have earned them. I feel the same way about my gray hairs too, which I will discuss in chapter 10, "Fifty Shades of Gray . . . Hair."

It is very important to acknowledge that midlife skin changes are really not *just* cosmetic. If our eyes are the windows into our soul, then our skin is the sliding screen door into our years of lifestyle choices. If you have not lived a healthy life, it will show up right on your face. Furthermore, how we look on the outside definitely affects how we feel on the inside, and vice versa. So let's get serious, without crinkling our brow, about what we can do to prevent, protect, and maintain the skin we have now.

SKIN IS NOT JUST SKIN DEEP

The skin is our largest organ and has many important jobs. It protects us against infection, dehydration, and physical damage from the sun. It also regulates our body temperature and turns sunlight into vitamin D, which is essential for healthy bones, as you will read in chapter 14, "Sticks and Stones Can Break Your Bones."

Skin is made up of three main layers. Starting from the top, there is the epidermis, followed by the dermis in the middle, and down at the bottom is the hypodermis. Tucked inside the epidermis are melanocytes, which are cells that produce melanin, a protective brown pigment that leads to a tan. Melanin shields the deeper layers of the skin from the harmful effects of the sun. The middle dermis layer forms the main bulk of the skin and is made up of proteins called collagen and elastin. Collagen is responsible for strength, structure, and firmness. Elastin maintains elasticity.

YOUTH IS WASTED ON THE YOUNG

When we age, our skin undergoes profound changes in all the layers. These result in decreased thickness, firmness, and elasticity, and increased wrinkles, sagging, and dryness. In fact, the biggest complaint that I hear from my patients is how dry their skin has become. It seems like all of a sudden, women go from soft and smooth to all dried up without so much as a warning bell. You have probably also noticed that along with thinner, more fragile skin comes more bruising when you bump into things. And to make matters even worse, the fat content of our skin decreases with age too. This will leave us looking saggy and probably make many of us feel like an old sad sack. If only the fat content decreased from our middle, muffin-top area instead. Please review chapter 7, "What's the Skinny on Weight Gain?"

HERE COMES THE SUN

When flipping through magazines, have any of you ever noticed the beautiful women in bathing suits basking in the golden sunshine on a tropical island? That looks very appealing. Every time I see this, I fantasize about hopping on a flight to the Caribbean. Now I want you to notice the advertisement that follows about two pages later, touting the latest age-defying skin cream to reduce fine lines and wrinkles. Those smart Mad Men are purposefully trying to get us to sit in the sun, and then buy cream to fix the sun damage!

We are all from that Coppertone generation, when women slathered on globs of tanning oil and perched in front of a silvery sun reflector thingamabob in order to get extra crispy. I can still at delicious coconut fragrance of summer. I can also still recall the pain of that first terrible sunburn. If we only knew then what we definitely know now about the harmful effects of the sun on skin health and wellness. No matter how golden brown you get from a tan, it really only means that your melanocytes are hard at work trying to protect you from the ravages of the sun. And the best reason of all to avoid too much sun exposure is to protect yourself from skin cancer.

So this is where I have to play the heavy when it comes to your complaints of skin changes in midlife. If you are serious about protecting the health of your skin, your days of lying out in the sun are now over. Not only that, you will have to apply sunscreen every single day of the year. Sunscreen is not just for summer anymore. My favorite is Neutrogena Ultra Sheer Dry-Touch Broad Spectrum SPF 30. I never leave home without it. In addition to your face and neck, don't forget to cover your ears, décolletage, and the backs of your hands. I am only reminding you of these additional areas because most of you have indeed forsaken them over the years. V-neck shirts are out too. Cover-ups and caftans are in.

By the way, you will never, ever find me lying out in the sun. Instead, what you will see is a middle-aged woman covered from head to toe in sun-protective clothing, wearing a large sombrero and enormous sunglasses and sitting underneath the shade of a beach umbrella. I won't care if you laugh at me. I definitely do not look sexy at the beach. But my healthy skin and I are totally okay with any snickering. I would also like to mention that because I am so careful about sun exposure, I have subsequently blocked my skin's ability to synthesize vitamin D. Since I would rather have lovely skin and avoid skin cancer, I take a daily vitamin D supplement in order to get my requirement for bone health.

Skin Protection Secrets

» Avoid the strong midday sun.
» Apply sunscreen with SPF 30 daily.
» Invest in a gorgeous wide brimmed hat.
» Never leave home without sunglasses.
» Wear sun-protective clothing.
» Stop sunbathing.
» Skip tanning salons.

QUIT SMOKING, FOR GOD'S SAKE!

Despite my best counseling efforts, I still have patients who continue to smoke cigarettes. I spend a lot of time discussing the most serious consequences of smoking, like heart disease, cancer, and stroke. When that fails, I hit women right in the vanity chops! That is when I lay down the argument for beautiful skin and remind women of the damage that smoking causes. I will often joke that if they cannot quit for themselves, they should quit for me. Then I can stop nagging them every year.

WHAT'S MENOPAUSE GOT TO DO WITH IT?

Estrogen plays a vital part in the health and wellness of our skin. It is important for preserving collagen and elastin as well as maintaining skin moisture and thickness. Best of all, it reduces skin wrinkles and improves blood supply. During the first five years of menopause, women can lose as much as 30 percent of our skin collagen. You may have also noticed that it takes longer for a skin cut to heal or a bruise to fade. That's because estrogen is critical for wound healing too. By the way, as you will learn in chapter 14, "Sticks and Stones Can Break Your Bones," this time period coincides with rapid bone loss. All heck seems to be breaking loose during these early menopausal years.

There is absolutely no doubt that estrogen therapy is beneficial when it comes to skin health. And we should not have to downplay the role that beautiful skin plays in improving our self-esteem, confidence, and overall quality of life. The only wrinkle here is that the FDA has not approved estrogen therapy use for these skin benefits. So what. If you are choosing hormone therapy to manage your menopause symptoms, you will also enjoy this added bonus of healthier and more youthful skin.

A WRINKLE IN TIME

As you will read in chapter 21, "Your Story," I love women who smile a lot. The only downside to smiling are wrinkles. Frowning and squinting cause wrinkles too. So if you want to decrease the lines in your forehead, the ridges above your nose, and the crow's-feet leaving footprints all around your eyes, then the first thing to do is stare blankly into space at all times. If that is not practical, then at least frown and squint less.

That reminds me of a story. I enjoy a rigorous spin class. At some point, I began to notice all the women around me getting really into the workout. As they were huffing and puffing and grunting their way to cardiac nirvana, they were also scrunching up their faces. That is when I had an Oprah aha! moment. I started mentioning to all my cycling classmates to relax their faces in order to stave off wrinkle formation. I'm sure some of them thought I was a little bit crazy. If you ever see me in class, though, check out my face. Although I am killing it on the bike, my face is the picture of serenity.

THE FRUITS AND VEGETABLES OF ETERNAL YOUTH

There is plenty of scientific evidence to support the fact that a healthy diet is good for your skin too. The antioxidants found in fruits, vegetables, and olive oil protect skin from the damaging effects of oxidative stress caused by sun exposure. At this point in *Menopause Confidential*, you already know that every fruit and vegetable has made the cut for healthy eating. So go cut up some celery sticks and eat your way to gorgeous skin.

AN OUNCE OF PREVENTION AND THEN
A POUND OF TREATMENT

It's never too late to adopt a skin-protective healthy lifestyle, even if you're already noticing the effects of aging, sun damage, cigarette smoking, and poor nutrition. For those of you who want to take wrinkle removal a step further, I have listed some common treatment options that are offered by dermatologists and plastic surgeons.

> **Wrinkles Begone!**
>
> » Topical glycolic acid
> » Retinoids
> » Chemical peels
> » Botox
> » Fillers
> » Laser resurfacing
> » Minimally invasive surgery

SPOT ON, SPOT OFF

Many midlife women develop brown age spots on their face and hands. These are sometimes referred to as liver spots, although the liver has nothing to do with them. We can blame the sun for these changes in skin texture and pigmentation. I am mentioning this to you now as a reminder that you should definitely have a dermatologist look at all of your moles, growths, and spots once a year to make sure none is precancerous or cancerous.

A leopard cannot change its spots, but we can. There are several over-the-counter topical preparations available for removing or lightening age spots. These creams are not as powerful as prescription remedies and will take at least six months before you will notice a modest improvement. For those of you who want to take spot removal a step further, I have listed some common treatments offered by dermatologists and plastic surgeons.

Out, Damned Spot!

» Retinoids
» Hydroquinones
» Intense pulsed light therapy
» Cryotherapy
» Laser resurfacing

ACNE AT *MY AGE*?

Acne is terrible at any age, but it always comes as such a surprise to women when it occurs at midlife. It is caused by a change in the balance of our hormones. Although estrogen is on the decline, testosterone, the pimple culprit, is still being produced by our semi-retired ovaries. At least 25 percent of you are going to experience acne during the menopausal transition. Interestingly, if you had acne as a teenager, you are more likely to have it as a grown-up.

As you will learn in chapter 16, "Potions, Patches, and Pills, Oh My!," if you are in the throes of perimenopause, a low-dose birth control pill will help improve acne. And if you are officially in the Menopause Club, your testosterone production will taper off about five years after you wave good-bye to your last menstrual period. So over time, your face will most likely become clearer all by itself.

For those of you who are suffering with severe adult acne, you will have to consult with a dermatologist for the latest treatment options available.

MY SKIN CARE REGIMEN

At the risk of sounding like a walking advertisement for specific skin care products, I thought it might be helpful to share my own daily skin health routine. I try to use common sense, and then I keep it simple and inexpensive. At bedtime, I always remove my makeup with Neutrogena cleansing towelettes. Then I wash my face with Cetaphil facial cleanser and moisturize with Neutrogena Triple Age Repair. About three times a week, I break out my pink Clarisonic PLUS scrubbing brush to exfoliate dead facial epidermal cells. That is my favorite glowy face secret. I also absolutely love Nivea body lotion and generously slather it all over after a shower. I can still sing the jingle from their 1970s commercial. And after a luxurious bath, there is nothing better than Neutrogena Body Oil with the light sesame fragrance.

In the morning, I splash my face with lukewarm water and apply Neutrogena sunscreen to my face, my neck, and the back of my hands. And don't forget about your lips. I cannot say enough nice things about Badger Lavender and Orange Lip Balm. I also love the round and colorful eos lip balms, because they are so easy to spot at the bottom of a crowded handbag.

ANOTHER BIG REVEAL

It wasn't until I turned fifty that I began to notice *and* be bothered by my own droopy eyelids, deepening grooves between my brows, marionette lines extending from my nose to my mouth, and jowls hanging down on either side of my chin. I am exaggerating to make the point that despite the fact that eyesight worsens with age, we see our own flaws clearly and in ten-times magnification.

Prior to that milestone birthday, I had absolutely no intention whatsoever of engaging in any cosmetic skin procedures. But a girl can change her mind, and so I did. In the spirit of full disclosure, I want you to know that I have sparingly tried Botox and fillers. I prefer to look natural, so I do not use these treatments often.

However, my bigger secret is that I did undergo surgery to un-droop my droopy eyelids. Believe me when I say that I did not make this decision lightly. But my lids had gotten so heavy that I began to have trouble keeping my eyes open. I have not shared this secret with my own patients yet. You are the first to know.

CHAPTER 10

Fifty Shades of Gray . . . Hair

I don't have gray hair. I have wisdom highlights.

—ANONYMOUS

MY QUEENDOM FOR A beautiful and full head of hair! Thinning and loss are common complaints during the menopause transition. Many of you have experienced a change in hair texture too. Instead of soft and silky, you've got rough and wiry, like a Brillo pad. But wait, there's more. Some midlife women are actually getting hairier, which can be scarier. That's because it is in all the wrong places, like on the face and chest. An unlucky few of you will experience both. And let's talk about all those gray hairs. I am rather proud of mine, but I know that many of you feel differently. Finally, we can no longer ignore the fact that our nails have become cracked and brittle too. All this bad news is enough to make you want to pull your hair out. But that would be a mistake. As you will soon learn, it takes years to grow a hair.

Needless to say, hair health is one of the most important issues for women of any age. However, it is particularly prickly for women in midlife as we face the loss of our youthful allure. Let's not minimize the importance of our gorgeous goldy locks. As you have learned in chapter 9, "Who Is That Wrinkly Old Woman in the Mirror?," our appearance is a reflection of overall health and wellness.

THE LIFE CYCLE OF A HAIR

Each hair develops from a follicle, which is a little pocket in the skin. Growth occurs in three phases. The first is an active growth phase, which lasts from two to six years. Next comes a quickie two-week transition phase. That's when the hair starts to make its way to the surface of the skin in preparation for the final resting phase. After a nice three-month rest, the hair falls out. This is the annoying moment when you see it on your hairbrush or clogging up the shower drain. Then the circle of hair life begins all over again.

The portion of hair that sticks out of your skin is called the hair shaft. The outermost part of the shaft is the cuticle. Its job is to strengthen and protect the shaft. Each strand of hair is constructed from proteins called keratins, which form the central core of the shaft and cuticle. Keratin gives the strand pliability. A balance of protein and moisture is necessary to maintain healthy hair. Maybe that's why advertisers are always trying to sell us bottles of moisturizing shampoo that claim they are filled with protein and keratin.

HAIR TODAY, GONE TOMORROW

At some point in life, one-third of women will experience *alopecia,* which is the medical term for hair loss. And about two-thirds of midlife women will suffer from hair thinning or bald spots. Women rarely become completely bald.

Female pattern hair loss (FPHL) is the most common cause and typically occurs gradually. The mechanism for this loss may have something to do with the imbalance of hormones that occurs when we join the Menopause Club. But genetics, lifestyle choices, stress, thyroid disease, certain medications, and the unknown play a part too.

THE ROLE OF HORMONES

As with practically every other bit of our womanly bodies, estrogen receptors are found in hair follicles too. And while the precise mechanism of action of estrogen is not known, estrogen is thought to prolong the growth phase of the hair cycle.

You already have a sense of this menopause connection, because your hair thinning or hair loss issues usually occur after your final menstrual period, when your ovaries have hit retirement. And for those of you who choose estrogen therapy for the treatment of your menopause symptoms, you also happily report an overall improvement in the health of your hair.

Testosterone plays a role here too. It gets converted to dihydrotestosterone (DHT) within the follicle, which leads to a reduced hair growth phase. That leads to shorter, thinner, and more brittle strands of hair as well as delayed growth of new hair. There is also a decrease in the total number of follicles. And, depending on the body area, DHT can either cause hair loss or unwanted hair growth, due to the hormonal imbalance caused when estrogen declines.

A HAIR IS A TERRIBLE THING TO WASTE

Once you have sought the advice of a healthcare professional and ruled out medical conditions that contribute to hair loss, you will have to use your old-fashioned common sense when it comes to caring for your hair. Eat a healthy diet, get plenty of rest, be physically active, quit smoking, and handle your hair very gently. Use moisturizing shampoos and leave-in conditioners. Comb your delicate hair with care, and skip the hair dryer when possible. I wash my hair just two or three times a week and use only a wide-toothed comb. My secret hair tip is to massage in some Moroccanoil for extra moisture and sleekness.

Hair Loss Treatments (Some Off-Label)

» Minoxidil
» Spironolactone
» Finasteride
» Estrogen therapy
» Low-energy laser light brush
» Hair transplantation

BEWARE OF CHIN HAIR

Hirsutism is a term used to describe hair growth in a typically male pattern location, such as the chin, upper lip, face, arms, lower abdomen, and inner thighs. Back in Barnum & Bailey's circus heyday, the Bearded Lady was sadly suffering from hirsutism. Scary witches always have one long, coarse hair growing out of a mole on their chins. You will never see any facial hair on Glinda, the Good Witch.

When hirsutism occurs in midlife, the cause is usually due to the same hormone imbalance that is also responsible for adult acne, with estrogen on the downswing and testosterone still kicking around. However, other common hair-raising conditions should be ruled out, like diabetes, thyroid disease, and adrenal hyperplasia. The management of midlife hirsutism combines mechanical depilation and prescription medication.

Ways to Remove the Strays

- » Plucking
- » Waxing
- » Shaving
- » Bleaching
- » Depilatory cream
- » Electrolysis
- » Laser therapy

Off-Label Prescriptions

- » Birth control pills
- » Spironolactone
- » Finasteride

GRAY, GRAY, GO AWAY

The main causes of graying hair are age, genetics, and lifestyle. Menopause has nothing to do with it. Just like in our skin, hair follicles have melanocytes that produce melanin. As you'll recall from chapter 9, "Who Is That Wrinkly Old Woman in the Mirror?," melanin is responsible for pigment. We make less melanin when we get older. So, over time, our hair color just fades to gray. Genetics play a very strong role in the graying of America. If one of your parents went prematurely gray, your head has a good chance of following in those footsteps. As far as lifestyle factors go, stress, smoking, obesity, chronic illness, and a poor diet have all been associated with accelerating your trip to Grayville.

AN OLD WIVES' TALE

I am very fond of that expression. Perhaps it is because I am now an old wife myself. I always joke that there are a lot of old wives out there telling tales. Here is one of my favorites. Does plucking your gray hair cause more to sprout? Nope. Each hair follicle grows only one hair. When you pluck it out, a new hair will grow back. It will take years to grow, as you now know. And it will still be gray. Be mindful that plucking can damage a hair follicle. So if you do a lot of plucking, don't be surprised when all the old wives start clucking about your new bald spot.

THE LIFE CYCLE OF A NAIL

Nails grow throughout life. Fingernails grow faster than toenails, but the whole process is still very slow. On average, it takes close to six months to replace a fingernail and over a year to replace a toenail. We reach peak nail health in our thirties, and then it starts to go downhill from there.

Many midlife women complain about changes in their nails. Have you noticed that yours are thinner, cracking, peeling, chipping, more brittle, or yellowing? That is not a coincidence, of course. Your nail health takes a dramatic dip after the age of fifty. It is not clear what role estrogen plays here. But knowing estrogen the way we do now, it certainly must have something to do with protecting our nail health.

Nails are made up of keratin, water, fat, iron, zinc, and calcium. Keratin is responsible for hardness and strength. The varying levels of water and fat keep our nails hydrated and moisturized. The nail bed underneath the nail contains tiny blood vessels and melanocytes, responsible for color. After menopause, the fat and water content decline. The blood supply dwindles and the aging melanocytes change up the nail color. All of that leads to dry and brittle nails, which are prone to cracking, pitting, yellowing, and the development of ridges and striations.

BE KIND TO YOUR FINGERS AND TOES

To maximize your nail health, make sure to eat a healthy diet rich in iron, zinc, and calcium. Avoid anything that can dry nails out, like the sun and harsh nail polish remover. Wear protective gloves when doing household cleaning chores, and be kind to your cuticles.

When I was ten years old, my Nana bought me a manicure kit. From that day on, I mastered the art of the manicure. I estimate that Nana has saved me swillions of dollars in manicure money, since I always do my own. I am very careful when cutting and filing my nails. And I moisturize my cuticles and nails every day with Sally Hansen cuticle oil. I love to joke that if my doctor career does not work out for me, I could easily open up my own nail shop. As a word of caution to you, if you would like to continue to enjoy the luxury of getting your nails groomed at your local salon, at least bring along your own manicure tools, for better safety and cleanliness, and ask the technician to be gentle.

MIRROR, MIRROR, ON THE WALL

Midlife women are the fairest of them all! Well, that may not be altogether true. However, I happen to think we are pretty great, even when we are having a bad hair day or have chipped a nail.

So when it comes to hair and nail health, let's do our best to choose a healthy lifestyle, seek professional help when necessary, and remember that inner beauty really is as important as all those old wives told us when we were young and full of hair-brained ideas.

As an aside, when my daughter was younger, she asked me if she was a princess. I told her that she definitely was, because her mother was a queen! I want you to feel the same way about yourself. Now, go and moisturize your feet.

CHAPTER 11

It's All About the Breast

I cannot believe they haven't come up with a
better screening process than the mammogram. If
a man had to put his special parts inside a clamp
to test him for anything, I think they would come
up with a new plan before the doctor finished
saying, "Put that thing there so I can crush it."

—ELLEN DEGENERES

IN MY CLINICAL EXPERIENCE, there is almost nothing that midlife
women fear more than breast cancer. Since breast cancer ranks second to lung cancer (listen up, smokers!) as the leading cause of cancer death affecting women over the age of forty, there is good reason
for concern, right? Well, let me put the fear of breast cancer into
perspective, so we can all spend less time worrying and more time
living healthy, meaningful, and fearless lives.

Every year, approximately 230,000 women are diagnosed with breast cancer and about 40,000 will die from the disease. As you can see from these numbers, the vast majority of women diagnosed with breast cancer will not die. In fact, they will live full lives and die from something else. How about some more good news? Despite what you have heard, the risk of breast cancer is low for women in their forties. As a result of this fact, mammography recommendations have recently changed for these youngsters. It is all very confusing, but do not dismay. I will sort it all out for you now.

Breast cancer screening guidelines were updated in 2015. And like cervical cancer screening, detailed in chapter 13, "The Latest Rap About the Pap," yet another women's health issue was brought to the forefront, inciting confusion, protest, anger, and suspicion that women's breasts do not matter to the mysterious people who are responsible for creating guidelines. Let me reassure you that the experts involved in reviewing the best available scientific information about breast cancer screening are really on our side. They are not just arbitrarily revising guidelines. For women to get the most up-to-date care, it is very important to periodically revisit older recommendations in light of new and better information. And you can take comfort in knowing that the current evidence-based guidelines were derived without any consideration to insurance coverage, legal issues, or cost.

The updated recommendations under the most scrutiny at the moment are those for a specific group of women: *average risk* forty-somethings. However, all the rest of us will be facing some new choices too. Most women are at average risk for breast cancer. If you have any breast cancer risk factors, these new guidelines do not apply to you.

It turns out that annual screening mammography in this

younger, premenopausal age group is no longer being universally recommended, because the best scientific information currently available does not support that women in their forties will benefit as much as was previously thought. Additionally, these younger women are more likely to suffer harm from the screening mammogram. I know this will surprise you, so I'll explain. First, though, let's back up a bit so you understand why mammograms have become such a hot-button issue.

Breast Cancer Risk Factors

» Dense breasts
» Early menses
» Later childbearing
» Abnormal breast biopsies
» Family history
» BRCA gene mutation
» Chest radiation

A HISTORY LESSON

Mammography has been around for over a hundred years and has saved many lives through the early detection of breast cancer. In 1913, a German surgeon was the first to use X-rays to look inside breasts for abnormalities. Around 1949, a radiologist from Uruguay introduced the dreaded breast compression technique. So for all of you who have suffered mightily while getting your breasts squeezed and flattened out like pancakes, at the same time wondering aloud if it was a man who developed that technique, your instincts were correct. Although we should all thank him for helping to save lives by improving the quality of mammographic screening, grateful is not the feeling we have when our breasts are being squashed in the cold metal vise grip as we hold both our breath and our tears. I usually tell the technician compressing my breasts that she is a torturer. I will apologize to her next time.

By the mid-1960s, mammography's early-detection capability was scientifically proven to reduce breast cancer death by 15 to 20 percent, and therefore took its rightful place in history as a great boon to women's health. In 1969, the modern-day film mammogram was invented. By 2000, film mammography was replaced with digital technology, which reminds me of the same fate that befell my beloved little Kodak camera. In 2011, 3-D mammography, also called breast tomosynthesis, was introduced with a grand claim that it was superior to the digital system. The jury is still out on whether this is true. Nevertheless, we have really come a long way from the original technology that started us out on the road to breast cancer screening.

However, for those of you who are wondering if there has been any headway made to eliminate the need for the breast squeeze-and-flatten technique, I am sorry to say that we are still stuck with it for the time being. Who among you is willing to invent something more comfortable?

THE NEW BREAST CANCER SCREENING GUIDELINES

Every few years, the recommendations regarding the who, what, when, where, and why women should get mammograms change.

Our first instinct is to blame the insurance companies for not wanting to pay up. Our next response is to ignore any new guidelines completely. And finally, we look to our healthcare professional for advice on what to do. Unfortunately, many of them are confused too. I receive many e-mail inquiries from my patients about whether or not they should keep their annual mammogram appointments. Remember, the goal of screening tests is to find disease early and not cause harm in the process. Let me sort out the latest breast cancer screening guidelines once and for all . . . until they change again!

Did You Know?

More than 50 percent of women who develop breast cancer have no known risk factors.

For most average risk women, the old guidelines were simple and easy to follow. Get your first mammogram at the age of thirty-five to establish a baseline picture. Then, starting at forty, get one every year forevermore. The rationale has always been that early detection of breast cancer through mammographic screening saves lives. However, after an extensive and careful review of the scientific literature and a better understanding of how breast cancer behaves among different ages and menopausal status, more fine-tuned recommendations have emerged.

Despite the fact that younger women, and by that I mean women under the age of fifty, are at an inherently lower risk for breast cancer, all breast cancers are not created equal. The ones that are diagnosed in younger women are usually more aggressive and deadlier than the ones discovered in women over fifty, who are likely already menopausal or well on their way. That's because younger women have denser breast tissue and are still making plenty of estrogen, both of which increase breast cancer risk. Denser breast tissue also makes mammography less helpful in detecting cancer in the first place.

That women under age fifty develop faster-growing, deadlier cancers than their older counterparts may make it seem all the more important for them to get mammograms. But it turns out that, even aside from the fact that mammography is less useful for detecting cancer in younger breasts, data show that the number of women in that age group who avoid dying from breast cancer through early detection is very small. In other words, the mammographic screening in younger women does not appear to significantly improve the outcome of finding these inherently deadlier tumors. What's more, women in this age group have a higher risk of being diagnosed and treated for *noninvasive* breast cancer.

On the other hand, most women over fifty-five, especially those who have transitioned through menopause, have less dense breasts and no longer make estrogen from their ovaries, so they are less likely to have a fast-growing or aggressive cancer. That is good news, since the majority of women who are diagnosed with breast cancer fall into this group. If you happen to be diagnosed with breast cancer after menopause, at least you can feel less worried that it will lead to your untimely death. The same cannot be said for heart disease, however, as you will learn in chapter 15, "I Left My Heart in San Francisco." To quote the legendary film star Bette Davis, "Old age ain't no place for sissies!"

WEIGHING BENEFIT AGAINST HARM

The mammogram debate really all boils down to who will benefit from early detection, because it has translated into a decreased
risk of *dying* from breast cancer versus who will be harmed by early
detection due to needless medical intervention. Will your mammogram find early cancer and save your life? Or will it find something
that ultimately leads to nothing after you have had additional invasive follow-up testing and several unnecessary, potentially painful
biopsies?

Even worse, could screening lead to *overdiagnosis*? That means
a breast cancer is indeed found and subsequently treated with surgery, chemotherapy, and radiation when, had everything been left
alone, your breast cancer would never have grown and caused any
problems at all. Putting your health in jeopardy through surgery,
suffering the side effects of radiation and chemotherapy, and living
with a fear of dying fall squarely into the harm category.

A Look at the Numbers

If you screen 1,900 women ages 40–49 . . .
» 1,000 women will have false alarms.
» 1 life will be saved.

Harm versus benefit is also currently part of the debate surrounding the diagnosis of ductal carcinoma in situ (DCIS), which
is the presence of noninvasive cancer cells in the milk ducts. This
type of cancer is determined by biopsy and usually found in younger

breasts. Think of DCIS cells as straddling a fence. They may cross over to the cancer side and become invasive many years from now. However, there is a greater likelihood that they will *not* cross over. Many a woman has lived to a ripe old age with DCIS. However, for those of you who might fall into this category, whether or not to take action is a tough decision. The additional harm includes your perception of being a ticking time bomb if these preinvasive cancer cells should grow. We can all understand how that would affect your feelings about your health, relationships, and overall quality of life.

I want you to really understand the important medical concept of harm versus benefit. If doing a test does not change the outcome of your disease, why do the test? Furthermore, if doing the test results in your having more tests, surgery, chemotherapy, and radiation while not changing the outcome of your disease, what was the point of it all? Remember that screening tests have to strike a reasonable balance between benefit and harm. In the case of mammographic screening for younger women, the risk of unnecessary breast biopsies and overdiagnosis appears to be higher than the benefit, especially because younger women are at a lower risk of breast cancer in the first place.

Younger breasts are filled with many interesting looking things. All of that interest leads to more false alarms requiring more biopsies that leave scars on beautiful breasts that should never have been biopsied at all. And that is the whole story in a nutshell.

WHY CAN'T EVERYONE AGREE?

There is a lot of disagreement among experts regarding forty-somethings. The American College of Obstetricians and Gynecologists

(ACOG) still recommends annual mammography starting at the age of forty. On the other hand, the United States Preventive Services Task Force (USPSTF), a volunteer panel of independent national experts, says that women should start mammography at the age of fifty and repeat it every other year instead of annually. The recently updated guidelines set forth by the American Cancer Society (ACS) seem to have split the difference by recommending that women start annual screening at the age of forty-five. Are you following all of this?

I am, by the way, going to argue for the other side of this issue shortly, having honed my debating skills while watching presidential candidates duke it out on TV.

BREAST DENSITY MATTERS

Before I talk about the other side of the mammogram issue, let me introduce a factor that also warrants consideration. Besides looking for breast cancer, mammography also detects differences in breast tissue density. That is important, because women with dense breasts have an increased risk of breast cancer and may require further imaging in the form of a breast ultrasound.

Breast density comes in four varieties: fatty, scattered fibroglandular, heterogeneously dense, and extremely dense. Mammography is more accurate when your breasts are almost entirely fatty. Isn't that ironic? We spend a lot of time worrying about getting fat, and it turns out to be fabulous when it comes to visualizing breast tissue!

Scattered fibroglandular is a mix of some dense tissue along with fat. Mammography is pretty good at seeing clearly in this breast tissue, although it can still miss a cancer hiding out in the dense area. Heterogeneously dense and extremely dense breasts render the mammogram much less effective, and 40 percent of women over forty will fall into these last two categories. So if your mammogram report states that you have either one of these diagnoses, you have dense breasts and are at increased risk for breast cancer. But take heart, increased risk does not mean it is a foregone conclusion. The good news is that most women with dense breasts will never develop cancer.

Sometimes doctors recommend other types of imaging for women who have dense breasts. Ultrasound sees things differently than mammograms; likewise magnetic resonance imaging (MRI). Surprisingly, though, there are currently no guidelines for all of you dense-breasted women regarding whether or not you should get a breast ultrasound or MRI. While breast ultrasound definitely helps find breast cancer that is missed by mammography, there is currently no scientific evidence that this finding will translate into a decrease in mortality. And that seems to be the bar by which breast cancer screening is set. As for breast MRIs, they are best reserved for women who are at high risk for breast cancer or who have already been diagnosed with the disease. They are not recommended for average risk women, because they lead to a lot of false alarms.

Extra, Extra

The risk of driving your car to get a mammogram might outweigh the benefits!

—*NEW YORK TIMES MAGAZINE*, MAY 1997

If all dense-breasted women decided to get breast ultrasounds, a thousand of us would then undergo breast biopsies, but only three or four breast cancers would be found. Now some of you may be willing to get additional ultrasound screening, knowing that it might lead to a breast biopsy that turns out to be nothing at all. And others of you may decide that since the overall additional risk of breast cancer in dense-breasted women is low, you would rather leave well enough alone. *There is no right answer.*

What I choose to do for my own dense breasts is get an ultrasound every other year. Although there is no science behind my strategy, it just seems to make the most sense to me.

LET THE DEBATE BEGIN!

Now that you understand why there is so much confusion about who will benefit from screening mammography or additional imaging such as breast ultrasound, let me acknowledge those who vehemently disagree with the recent changes in the guidelines. Many radiologists, breast cancer surgeons, gynecologists, and women feel that it is preferable to continue screening women every year in order to find a smaller breast cancer at an earlier stage. This would allow for a simpler surgery and perhaps less need for chemotherapy and radiation, even if it does not change the ultimate outcome of dying. When you think about breast cancer in this way, it is not only about dying but also about living without having to endure major disfiguring surgery, chemotherapy, and radiation. And that brings us right back to the same issue of balancing benefit versus harm. If you are the kind of woman who prefers to stick with mammographic screening every year, regardless of any potential harm, then that is the right decision for you. On the other hand, if you feel that the potential for additional surveillance, unnecessary biopsies, and overdiagnosis are too high a price to pay given your average risk of breast cancer, then following the latest guidelines might be best for you.

HERE IS WHERE I STAND ON THE MAMMOGRAM

Women are very capable of making intelligent decisions about practically anything once we have been presented with the pros and cons of the particular issue at hand. For all of you average risk women out there, I think that the American Cancer Society guidelines, outlined in the table on page 117, make the most medical sense and strike the best balance between benefit and harm.

Once you hit fifty-five, the screening interval changes to every other year. The rationale for the interval extension in this age group is that, as I mentioned earlier, breast cancer tends to grow more slowly and be less aggressive after menopause. Mammograms are also easier to interpret, since older breasts have a tendency to be less dense. So there is plenty of time to diagnose and treat women, while avoiding the extra surveillance, unnecessary biopsies, and overdiagnosis that result from screening too often.

THE GOLDEN GIRLS

What happens when you hit your so-called golden years? Well, according to the American Cancer Society, you have to be able to see into your future. When women ask me about health issues they may face down the road, I always lament that my crystal ball is broken. The best advice for now is that if you are healthy and think you've got another good ten years left, you should continue having mammograms every other year. On the other hand, if you think your clock is ticking faster than that, you can consider yourself a mammogram graduate and throw yourself a graduation party.

By the way, the USPSTF says that you can stop getting mammograms when you hit age seventy-five. So what should you do? Discuss this important decision with your healthcare professional.

CLINICAL AND SELF-BREAST EXAM HULLABALOO

Are you ready to be shocked? The American Cancer Society and the USPSTF have not found that a *clinical* breast exam, which is the one performed by a healthcare professional, adds any additional benefit over and above a mammogram when it comes to stomping out breast cancer. That means that your gynecologist will have even less to do during your annual visit if there is no need for a breast exam. And as you will soon learn in chapter 13, "The Latest Rap About the Pap," most of us do not need a Pap every single year either. Scandalous!

Now is the perfect time to reveal another secret. Believe it or not, there is absolutely no scientific evidence that doing your own monthly breast self-examination makes any difference whatsoever when it comes to diagnosing breast cancer early and affecting mortality rates later on. I know this sounds utterly blasphemous. When I first learned this information in 1990, I was an OB-GYN resident at the University of San Francisco, California. That was twenty-five years ago, and we are still teaching women to do breast self-exams. Why?

Despite the fact that breast self-exams do not save lives, they still serve a very important purpose. The point of doing them periodically is to find our own *normal.* We all have lumps and bumps, and the sooner we get comfortable with how they feel, the more informed we will be if anything changes. Remember that breasts do indeed change during our menstrual cycles, when they get even fuller and more tender to the touch. So take my advice and avoid doing your self-exams at that time of month. You will just find lots of lumps and bumps that will worry you.

If you choose to do a self-exam, the best time to do it is right after a menstrual cycle, when your breasts are the least stimulated and, therefore, less lumpy. This is also true for those of you with breast implants, which makes it harder to feel breast tissue. Do your best to feel around the edges of the implant and under your armpit. And don't bother doing self-exams every single month either. In fact, the American Cancer Society regards breast self-examination as something that is optional and to be done occasionally, rather than something essential to be performed monthly.

The truth of the matter is that by the time you can actually feel a cancerous lump in your own breast, it has been growing there for about ten years. And that means it has most likely spread to your lymph nodes and beyond, making it an advanced stage breast cancer. Here comes another secret. I never tell my patients to do regular self- breast examinations. I don't even do my own. Perhaps it's because women have enough to do, and I don't want to add one more thing that will feel like a homework assignment we are always forgetting. So if you feel like doing your own exam, go right ahead. And if you do not, that is fine too.

The 2015 American Cancer Society Guidelines

40–44 years young	Mammography optional
45–54 years old	Annual mammography
55 and up	Mammography every other year
Good health and life expectancy more than 10 years	Mammography every other year or every year if you really want to
Clinical breast exam	Not helpful

BRCA GENE TESTING

Angelina Jolie, the movie star, director, and humanitarian, changed the face of women's health single-handedly when she revealed to the world that she carried a gene mutation that put her at high risk for breast and ovarian cancer. She shocked practically the whole nation when she underwent two separate surgeries to have her breasts, ovaries, and fallopian tubes removed in order to significantly reduce her own risk. By telling her story, Angelina helped start an important conversation about who is at higher risk for these specific cancers and needs genetic testing. As it turns out, not all of us do. In fact, most of us don't.

Here comes another history lesson. There are two main genes responsible for increasing the risk of breast and ovarian cancer. BRCA1 was identified in 1994 and BRCA2 in 1995. We all carry these normal genes. Their role is to repair cell damage and make sure that breast and ovarian cells grow normally. But if either gene has a mutation, breast and ovarian cells can grow abnormally and transform into cancer.

Mutations tend to be passed down from generation to generation, increasing the risk of these cancers in certain families, especially of Eastern European Jewish descent. This mostly affects women, but men can inherit this gene and get breast cancer too. When considering your own risk, look into your family history to see if anyone has had a diagnosis of either breast or ovarian cancer, especially at a younger age. These cancers tend to present themselves when women are in their midthirties and forties, and they generally are aggressive. The good news is that only 1 to 2 percent of us have inherited this gene mutation. That means that 98 percent of us don't have to worry about genetic testing, because we don't have a higher risk of breast and ovarian cancer due to a genetic inheritance.

For those of you with a personal or family history of breast or ovarian cancer at an early age, I recommend genetic counseling to determine whether genetic testing is warranted. The BRCA blood test costs $3,000 and is not always covered by insurance. So if you don't need testing, you should not get it. If it turns out that you are indeed positive for either BRCA1 or BRCA2, you are at high risk for both breast and ovarian cancer. Thanks to Angelina Jolie, it is now much easier to have the difficult conversation about what comes next regarding the surgeries potentially required to reduce your risks. My best advice is to include an expert in menopausal medicine in the discussion, so you are fully informed about your choices for dealing with the symptoms of surgical menopause. In my own practice, I strongly recommend that women undergoing the removal of their ovaries and fallopian tubes have their uterus removed too. It will make using hormone therapy for the treatment of surgical menopause symptoms so much easier and safer.

WE ARE WOMEN, HEAR US ROAR!

I am thrilled to report that most of us will *not* be diagnosed with breast cancer. For those of us who will, this diagnosis is no longer the death sentence it used to be due to all of the excellent treatment options available. So as it turns out, it's not all about the breast after all. We are much more than that. We are women from head to toe and everything else in between.

CHAPTER 12

Hooray for Colonoscopy!

You've got a song you're singing from your gut.
You want that audience to feel it in their gut.

—JOHNNY CASH

WHEN WOMEN TURN FIFTY, I think two things should happen. First, we should throw ourselves a party, go on a trip, or at the very least, mark this spectacular milestone with a nice dinner out. Then we should schedule a screening colonoscopy. If you've made it all the way to this chapter, you know that I am really not kidding!

Colon cancer is the third leading cause of cancer death in women, behind lung and breast cancer. Every year an estimated 25,000 of us will die from this disease, most likely because so many avoid getting screened. Prevention and early detection are the key to survival. The gold standard for both is colonoscopy. I can hear some of you groaning and gagging right now. That's because you have either personally experienced a very unpleasant bowel preparation or heard about someone else's awful tale of woe. Perhaps the entire notion of getting a colonoscopy is so off-putting that you have put it off every year since hitting the big 5-O. Well, I always tell my patients that having colon cancer is much worse than getting a colonoscopy. Then I ask them to do their screening as a birthday present to themselves. And if not for them, I say, "Do it for me, your favorite gynecologist!" That usually works.

Did You Know?

Ninety percent of colon cancer in women is diagnosed over the age of 50.

The American Cancer Society (ACS) and the U.S. Preventive Services Task Force (USPSTF) seem to be in agreement about guidelines for colon cancer screening for *average risk* women. What a relief after all the confusion and mayhem in the previous chapter, "It's All About the Breast." Start your screening at the age of fifty and continue every five to ten years until the age of seventy-five. After that, routine screening is not recommended. Another graduation party! However, if you fall into a *high risk* group, these guidelines do not apply to you. Consult with your favorite gastroenterologist for an individualized schedule.

Cancer Risk Factors You Cannot Control

» Personal history of colorectal cancer, adenomatous polyps, or inflammatory bowel disease
» Family history of colorectal cancer, adenomatous polyps, or hereditary colorectal cancer syndrome
» Diabetes
» Hispanic and black ethnicity
» Age over 50

Cancer Risk Factors You Can Control

» Cigarette smoking
» Excessive alcohol consumption
» Sedentary lifestyle
» Obesity
» High fat/low fiber diet
» Too much red or processed meat

THE INS AND OUTS OF COLONOSCOPY

As you know, the goal of screening is to reduce the number of people who die from colon cancer. Colonoscopy is considered the gold standard because it allows the gastroenterologist to see the entire length of the colon as well as perform a biopsy of anything that looks interesting. This gets accomplished with a colonoscope, which is a thin, tubelike instrument with a light and a lens at the end. It is inserted into the body through the rectum. Don't worry. You are given really groovy anesthesia before the procedure and won't feel a thing.

I observed my one and only colonoscopy procedure when I was in medical school. That was over twenty-five years ago, and I can still really remember the excitement of it all. The gastroenterologist really does have a cool job. Do I sound geeky? Imagine walking through a very long, dark, narrow, and twisty tunnel with only one small flashlight. You have to tread carefully as you navigate the sharp turns, and you never know what's lurking just around the corner. It is not my intention to make colonoscopy sound scary. On the contrary, I think every procedure is more like a treasure hunt. The *booty* turns out to be precancerous growths called adenomatous polyps. Removing them is the key to avoiding cancer down the road. It takes about ten years for these polyps to transform into cancer. That's why the recommended screening interval is every five to ten years.

Hooray!

Colonoscopy reduces colon cancer risk by 90 percent.

Colonoscopy will also find full-blown colon cancer if it's there. And if you follow the screening guidelines, you will have the best chance of finding cancer early and getting treatment sooner. Then you will live a long life and die from something else. Feel free to jump ahead to chapter 15, "I Left My Heart in San Francisco," to learn about the number one killer of women in the United States.

Extra, Extra!

In 1990, a new kind of precancerous polyp called "serrated" was identified and found to be more common in women than in men.

THE DREADED BOWEL PREP EXPERIENCE
MADE ABSOLUTELY WONDERFUL

The only way for your gastroenterologist to do the best possible job for you is for *you* to do the best possible bowel preparation. You need to show up to your procedure squeaky-clean. When I turned fifty, I was very excited to schedule my first colonoscopy. Of course, I did not have the procedure done on my actual fiftieth birthday. Instead, I threw myself a disco dance party, followed by an adventure trip to the Galápagos Islands where I rubbed elbows with giant tortoises and blue-footed boobies. However, a month later, I found myself draped in a flimsy gown on a gurney awaiting my rite of passage. Coincidentally, a medical colleague of mine also happened to be getting her colonoscopy at the same surgery center, and we had a great time bonding before the moment of truth. I really wanted to win in the battle of the best bowel prep. And that is what I want for you too.

Without telling my gastroenterologist, I tweaked the instructions for the prep day because I felt confident that I could achieve the seemingly unachievable: a comfortable prep experience in addition to a complete clean-out. For those of you who do not yet know, the traditional bowel prep consists of drinking jugs of a really awful-tasting liquid laxative, which makes everyone feel lousy. The start time for this cocktail is usually set for late afternoon, which causes many of us to lose valuable sleep as we run to the bathroom for most of the night.

I am thrilled to report that not only was my prep day easy and efficient, allowing for an early bedtime, I also got an A+ from my doctor for my squeaky-clean colon. I have subsequently passed

along my secret recipe to my patients with great feedback and fan-
fare. Now I will share it with you.

MY SECRET RECIPE

You will need to purchase the following ingredients: Dulcolax suppositories, a bottle of seltzer water, two quarts of rich chicken con-
sommé, and Prepopik laxative powder, available by prescription only.

On prep day, you must avoid all solid foods as well as dark or
red liquids. First thing in the morning, start drinking your deli-
ciously warmed-up chicken broth, which is filled with fatty glob-
ules. Your brain will feel very satisfied, and your tummy will not
be hungry. Skip your usual morning cup of coffee, because it is a
dark liquid. Instead, insert *two* Dulcolax suppositories into your
rectum and await a bowel movement. That usually happens within
an hour. Repeat with two more rectal suppositories about three
hours later. Timing is important, because your colon does not like
to be rushed.

Following that second bowel movement, you will be practically
emptied out. The hard work is over, and it wasn't even all that hard!
Start your prescription laxative powder in the early afternoon. It
needs to be poured into a glass of clear liquid. I chose seltzer water
to make the whole experience fizzy and festive. Repeat with the second laxative powder packet in the early evening. What remains of
the day is the emergence of a darkish or yellowy liquidy poo and
some gas.

You should go to sleep by 10:00 PM and have a good night's rest.
Make sure you're on time for your appointment the next morning.

And always be nice to your nurses. If you don't get at least an A for squeaky-cleanness, please let me know immediately.

DO I REALLY NEED A COLONOSCOPY?

Yes, you really do. However, there are other screening tests available, if you are not able to get a colonoscopy. They include stool testing, flexible sigmoidoscopy, double-contrast barium enema, and a CT colonography. There are risks and benefits to all of these choices, so please have a discussion with your primary healthcare professional about what is right for you. If you want my opinion, however, I strongly recommend that, when possible, you always go with the gold standard.

REDUCE YOUR RISK

There are definitely some scientifically proven strategies you can incorporate into your daily life to reduce your risk of colon cancer. There are also many claims out there that have not panned out whatsoever. So let's stick with the ones that have panned in.

Physical activity has been credited with a 30 percent reduction in colon cancer risk. So put down this book, and let's get physical! A diet loaded with fruits, vegetables, and grains also appears to be protective, while one high in fat as well as red or processed meats puts you at risk. So please pass the broccoli and take a pass on the beef burrito.

The big news this year is that after decades of scientific study, it appears that low-dose aspirin, starting at the age of fifty and taken daily for at least ten years, is associated with a 20 to 40 percent reduction in both polyps and colon cancer. The USPSTF has recently released its official recommendation supporting low-dose aspirin use for the primary prevention of colon cancer. However, there are bleeding and ulcer risks associated with taking aspirin. So please ask your healthcare professional or favorite gastroenterologist whether or not you should take low-dose aspirin.

As for the vitamins and minerals C, D, E, B6, calcium, and folate in supplement form, there does not appear to be a strong association with colon cancer risk reduction, despite all the hubbub. It's better to get our vitamins and minerals from food sources than from tablets. That brings us right back to a healthy diet filled with fruits, vegetables, and grains. I think I shall order the lentil soup next time, with a spinach salad on the side.

BOTTOMS UP

I really enjoy sharing secrets with you, and here comes one about constipation! I always travel with Dulcolax suppositories. For some inexplicable reason, my colon almost never wants to poop in any other potty but its own at home. I know that happens to many of you too, so don't forget this valuable tip when packing for your fabulous fiftieth-birthday trip.

And of course, when it comes to colon cancer screening, don't fall behind or slip through the cracks! Sorry, I couldn't help myself.

CHAPTER 13

The Latest Rap About the Pap

Now what you hear is not a test,
I'm rappin' to the beat.

—THE SUGARHILL GANG

IN 2012, NEW CERVICAL cancer screening guidelines were published in the United States, making the traditional annual Pap a thing of the past. Instead, the newest guidelines recommend that the interval of cervical cancer screening be extended from annually to every three years if your previous test was normal.

This event shocked a nation of women, as well as their healthcare professionals. It completely upended the way women viewed the purpose of their annual gynecology visit. Why were women being deprived of a valuable yearly screening test that reduced the risk of cervical cancer? Was this a conspiracy by insurance companies to save money at the expense of women's health? What would gyne-cologists do all day, if they no longer had to perform Pap testing as frequently?

To make matters even worse, the new guidelines were so com-plicated and confusing that most healthcare professionals just ignored them and continued to encourage and perform annual Pap tests anyway. That approach seemed to be just fine with many women too, since 90 percent of you believe in the power of the Pap!

In 2014, I attended a lecture that would change my life. A renowned expert in the field of menopause told her audience to *demand* their Pap every year. I was shocked! I knew that was out-dated advice. Should I stay quiet and let all those women march around New York City insisting on unnecessary tests? It was at that very moment that I decided to write this book. And in case you were wondering, I also spoke out at the meeting in favor of the new guidelines. My remarks were *not* met with a standing ovation. In fact, the speaker actually yelled at me and told me I was wrong. Because of that life changing experience, I committed to writing a book based on the best scientific evidence currently available.

One of the central principles of medicine is "First do no harm." As it turns out, there are significant negative implications to *over*-screening for any disease. Recall the latest controversy surrounding the annual mammogram, as well as breast exams, in chapter 11, "It's All About the Breast." As we know, change is difficult. But the time has indeed come for us to change. So let's all take a collective deep breath, as I walk you through the latest rap about the Pap.

A HISTORY LESSON

In the early 1900s, cervical cancer was the number one killer of women in the United States. The good news is that cervical cancer is now considered rare in this country. That's because Dr. George Papanicolaou and his colleagues discovered that cervical cancer could be identified by inspecting cervical cells. Voilà! The Pap smear was invented. By the 1950s, it became the first screening test widely used for cancer detection. Today, approximately 13,000 women will be diagnosed with this disease and only 4,000 deaths will result. African American and Hispanic women have the highest rates of cervical cancer because statistically they are less likely to get Pap screening.

However, like most screening tests, the Pap smear has never been perfect. Over many decades, a lot of women have tested positive for abnormal cervical cells when, in fact, those cervical cells were perfectly normal. Those "abnormal" Pap smears led to additional biopsies and surgeries, causing both physical and psychological harm. At some point, it became clear that the more frequently women got Pap smears, the more false alarms they experienced.

I hesitate to point out the financial cost as well, lest you think that's the main motivation for decreased testing. However, let's all face the reality that choices must be made when it comes to spending our hard earned money on healthcare. Consider your own personal expenditures when going to a medical appointment. You have to take time off from work, arrange for child care, pay for parking, and usually wait for hours in a crowded room until it's your turn to be seen. Wouldn't it be preferable to do that only as often as you really needed to? The costs all add up.

A new, more accurate form of Pap test called liquid-based cytology was developed and introduced in 1996. That turned out to be much better than the traditional smear of yesteryear, and liquid-based cytology is what we use today. Many people still refer to this test as a Pap "smear." And even though this screening test is more accurate and better able to detect abnormal cervical cells, it is not a perfect test either.

THE CERVICAL CANCER MYSTERY IS SOLVED!

Around 1976, the human papillomavirus (HPV) was discovered to be the *actual cause* of cervical cancer. In fact, every cervical cancer starts out as an HPV infection. HPV is a sexually transmitted disease. The two most common high risk viral strains that lead to cervical cancer are HPV 16 and 18. However, there are at least a dozen more high risk culprits. There are also low risk strains of HPV, which are responsible for causing genital warts.

Extra, Extra!

Stockholm, Sweden, 2008

German virologist Harald zur Hausen wins the Nobel Prize for discovering HPV 16 and 18 in cervical cancer biopsies.

Congratulations, and thank you!

Now here comes another shocker! Most of us have been exposed to the HPV virus through sexual activity, and most of us can thank our immune systems for ridding our bodies of the HPV virus before it leads to infection and possibly cancer. This process of exposure and good riddance takes place over many years, and that is one of the reasons behind the extension of cervical cancer screening intervals. If we wait a few years, most problems will resolve all by themselves. Surprisingly, only a handful of you are aware of the HPV virus connection to cervical cancer. And even fewer of you have an understanding that most HPV infections go away on their own.

Another reason for the screening interval extension has to do with the fact that if we do indeed get an actual cervical infection that does not clear up, it takes several years to find it on a Pap test in the form of abnormal cervical cells called dysplasia, or precancerous changes. Then it takes about ten years for a small number of these cervical dysplasia cases to evolve into a cancer. So there really is plenty of time to detect abnormal cervical cells associated with high risk HPV virus strains long before the issue of cervical cancer rears its ugly head.

A brand new concept of *co-testing* with both Pap cytology and the HPV test was introduced between 2006 and 2009. The main advantage of co-testing is that women who test negative on *both* tests have practically no chance whatsoever of getting cervical cancer for years after that one screening. Years! So now you understand why it makes sense to extend the interval of cervical cancer screening from annually to every three years if your Pap test is normal, or every five years if your co-testing is normal.

Despite the fact that I explain all of this to my own patients, some still prefer to stick to the old regimen. Perhaps I am not doing a good enough job illuminating the harms of overtesting. For these reluctant-to-change women, I ease more slowly into the most current recommendations by extending the interval to every two years.

There is both an art and a science to the practice of medicine. It is important to be good at both. I do hope, though, I have made a clear and convincing argument for those of you who are still insisting on an annual Pap.

ROAD MAP THROUGH THE PAP

Let's take a moment to talk about the young people. HPV is especially common in sexually active teenagers and twenty-somethings. Because of this fact of life, we do not recommend HPV screening for them at all. Why not? It's because we know that we will find HPV and that most of these youngsters will clear the virus all by themselves over time. So the best thing to do is stay out of their private parts when it comes to looking for the virus. HPV screening starts when women turn thirty. Pap testing, however, begins at the age of twenty-one. If you happen to have tweenagers, you should definitely take them to their pediatrician for an HPV vaccination *before* they become sexually active. The vaccine is very effective in preventing infection from HPV 16 and 18.

How often should the Pap be repeated? Can you skip the Pap altogether and just do an HPV screen? What happens if you have a new sexual partner? Does that change the algorithm? What should you do if you have an abnormal Pap test or high risk HPV screen? Does cervical cancer screening go on forever?

As of 2013, the U.S. Preventive Services Task Force (USPSTF), the American Cancer Society (ACS), the American Society for Colposcopy and Cervical Pathology (ASCCP), and the American Society for Clinical Pathology (ASCP) have agreed to a recommendation for cervical cancer screening surveillance summarized below:

< 21 years old	No cervical cancer screening at all
21–29 years old	Pap every 3 years
30–65 years young	Pap every 3 years or co-testing with Pap and HPV every 5 years
65 and up	If you have had normal screening for the past 10 years, you are a graduate!
Women after hysterectomy	If your cervix has been removed and your surgery was not for cancer, you are a graduate!
HPV vaccinated	Guidelines remain the same
New sexual partner	Guidelines remain the same
HPV screening only	The jury is still out

If you happen to have an abnormal Pap test with moderate to severe cervical dysplasia or a positive high risk HPV screen, all of these recommendations go out the window. You will have to undergo further evaluation, called colposcopy, which is a high powered microscope aimed directly at your cervix. That exam will most likely lead to some cervical biopsies to determine if you really do have cervical dysplasia or cancer. Once you have been appropriately diagnosed, treated, and have normal follow-up testing, you can join the rest of the group again for routine screening.

LET'S RAP UP

I would like to share some closing thoughts about the importance of the annual GYN appointment. Despite the fact that we can and should extend our Pap test intervals if the previous screens have been *normal,* women are much more than just a cervix. There are so many other important health issues we will face, especially as we hit perimenopause and menopause. So now that we have found some extra time during the exam, let's use it wisely to focus on total body health and wellness. See you next year!

CHAPTER 14

Sticks and Stones Can
Break Your Bones

To succeed in life, you need three things: a
wishbone, a backbone, and a funny bone.

—REBA MCENTIRE

THE "STICKS AND STONES" childhood rhyme is my way of introducing the very adult topic of osteoporosis, a disabling disease characterized by thinning bones and reduced bone quality, leading to an increase in the risk of bone fracture. The management of osteoporosis in menopausal women is usually straightforward. The problem is that too few women are being properly screened and treated.

Menopausal women are at high risk for osteoporosis. Once we have stopped making our own estrogen, which is very protective of bone health, we rapidly lose bone, especially in the first few years after the menopause transition. This is the *most important* piece of information that you will get from this chapter. So you must start paying attention to improving your own bone health right now.

Have you ever noticed the older woman at the market who is completely hunched over? Her dowager's hump is caused by multiple vertebral compression fractures. My heart breaks every time I see a woman like this, because I know that osteoporosis is preventable in the first place, and treatable in the second. Do not allow yourselves to get to the hump stage!

Millions of women in the United States already carry the diagnosis of osteoporosis, as well as its less severe cousin, osteopenia, otherwise referred to as low bone mass. That means that there are millions of bone fractures happening every year. If you add them all up, they total more than breast cancers, hearts attacks, and strokes combined. Did you ever hear that before? I'll bet not. Perhaps it's because osteoporosis is often referred to as a *silent* disease. You only hear about it when you or your good friend has fractured a bone.

So let's break the silence, not our bones, once and for all. I want you to fear osteoporotic fractures as much as breast cancer and heart attacks. In fact, let's start thinking about bone fractures as *bone attacks* instead, and learn how to prevent the whole issue altogether. What can you do now to avoid joining the millions of women in the osteopenia and osteoporosis club?

Risk Factors You Cannot Control	Risk Factors You Can Control
» Female sex » Advanced age » White race » Personal history of fracture » Fracture in first degree relative » Dementia » Poor health » Fragility	» Eat a calcium-rich diet » Be physically active » Don't smoke » Don't drink too much alcohol » Maintain weight above 127 pounds » Be aware of medication side effects

RISKY BUSINESS

Age, genetics, and menopause play a big role in your personal risk, and you can't do much to change that. I always ask my patients if their mother is getting shorter, has the diagnosis of osteoporosis, or—even worse—has suffered a hip fracture. If your answer is "Yes" to any of those questions, consider yourself at higher risk. The menopause crowd is particularly vulnerable to bone loss, especially in the early years of the transition due to low estrogen levels. You're probably not being educated about the significant bone loss that occurs right at menopause. The *best* way for you to prevent osteoporosis and bone fracture is to prevent the bone loss that occurs during the menopause transition. You heard it here first!

Now there are a few risks that you can actually do something about to prevent osteoporosis and fracture later on. Please review the box titled "Risk Factors You Can Control" and decide what changes you can make today.

I am never sure what to recommend to the slim girls who weigh less than 127 pounds. You are at risk for this disease because of your thinness. Some of you were childhood gymnasts, ballerinas, or star athletes, and all that exercise had opposing effects. On the good side, you increased your bone mass. On the bad side, you may have skipped or stopped your menstrual cycles, which led to years of reduced bone protection from lack of consistent estrogen.

Some of you are just genetically thin, and it's not reasonable to suggest that you fatten up. Others of you are thin because you suffer from an eating disorder like anorexia nervosa, and that requires a much bigger conversation. No matter what the reason, you need to pay especially close attention to maximizing your bone health.

Common Medications That Cause Bone Loss

» Aromatase inhibitors
» Selective serotonin reuptake inhibitors (SSRIs)
» Proton pump inhibitors
» Steroids

I also want to give a specific shout-out to all the breast cancer survivors on aromatase inhibitors. You are at a higher risk for bone loss due to this medication. For some inexplicable reason, your group is not generally informed about this important issue. Aromatase inhibitors are necessary for the prevention of recurrent or new breast cancers, so you cannot stop taking them just to protect your bones. You need to be proactive and have a conversation with your healthcare professional about osteoporosis prevention.

STAY IN THE GAME

The diagnosis of osteoporosis is made either *after* you have already experienced a fracture, which is really too late, or by getting a screening dual-energy bone densitometry (DEXA) scan to see if your bone density measurements are sufficiently low to qualify for either osteopenia or osteoporosis. The DEXA report also includes a Fracture Risk Assessment Tool (FRAX) score, which is your ten-year risk assessment for getting a hip, spine, or forearm fracture. If your overall risk of fracture is 20 percent, or your hip-fracture risk is 3 percent, you will definitely need to get medical treatment. Game over.

We all should get a screening DEXA scan at the age of sixty-five, but many of us will need one sooner if we have risk factors. If your DEXA scan shows that you have lost enough bone to qualify for osteopenia or osteoporosis, it is generally repeated every two years. The reason for this long interval is that bone turnover is slow, and any changes that you make through improved lifestyle or medication will take time before an effect can be seen.

FRAX Factors

» Age
» Weight
» Height
» Current cigarette use
» Current alcohol use
» Parental hip fracture

» DEXA hip score
» Chronic use of steroids
» Rheumatoid arthritis
» Other causes of
   osteoporosis

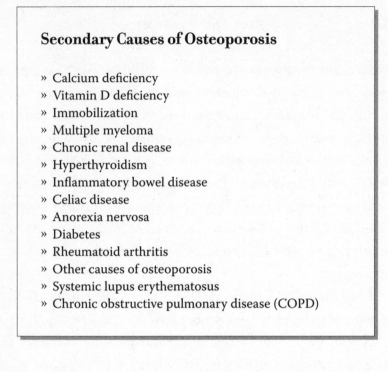

Secondary Causes of Osteoporosis

» Calcium deficiency
» Vitamin D deficiency
» Immobilization
» Multiple myeloma
» Chronic renal disease
» Hyperthyroidism
» Inflammatory bowel disease
» Celiac disease
» Anorexia nervosa
» Diabetes
» Rheumatoid arthritis
» Other causes of osteoporosis
» Systemic lupus erythematosus
» Chronic obstructive pulmonary disease (COPD)

LISTEN TO YOUR MOTHER!

Let's take a journey back to our childhood, when our mothers told us to drink milk. Dairy foods are a wonderful source of calcium, a mineral necessary for building and maintaining healthy bones. Momma's advice was very wise, because kids are actively building bone, especially at puberty, and need all the nutritional tools they can get in order to increase bone mass as well as strength. I always tell my patients to be a role model for their own sons and daughters when it comes to getting adequate calcium and vitamin D, especially during those key tween and teenage years. That goes for physical activity too, which you will learn all about in chapter 18, "Do I Really Have to Lift Weights Too?"

Figure out which foods you and your kids love that are rich in calcium and fortified with vitamin D, and eat more of those daily. A good rule of thumb is to make sure everyone gets two servings per day. I have recently begun warming up a cup of milk every night before bedtime for my own kids. Once our children reach their late twenties, they will have achieved peak bone mass. Sadly, it is all downhill from there in terms of bone acquisition. The best any of us can do after that is maintain, maintain, maintain! So don't squander a minute of your children's active bone building years. And since those same years often coincide with your menopause transition, this is great motivation for you to hitch a ride on the family bone health bandwagon! No more excuses.

Lest you think at your age that you have missed the boat on bone health, it is not too late to implement a bone strengthening lifestyle. It's a little-known fact that women can fracture a bone even when they are at the osteopenia stage. Many healthcare professionals do not take low bone mass seriously enough. Remember that old saying—"An ounce of prevention is worth a pound of cure." So let me offer up some useful ounces of prevention that we can all start today.

EAT AND DRINK YOUR CALCIUM AND VITAMIN D

There seems to be lots of confusion about how much calcium and vitamin D we should consume to keep our bones up and running. (Actually, I counsel against running, which is really very injurious to our aging bodies. Stay tuned, all you die-hard runners out there! More on that in chapter 18, "Do I Really Have to Lift Weights Too?") For now, let's talk about getting that all important calcium and vitamin D in.

Calcium Rich Foods

» Yogurt (my favorite: Chobani Coconut)
» Cheese
» Milk (my favorite: Skim Plus)
» Oranges
» Broccoli
» Kale
» Collard greens
» Bok choy
» Figs
» Canned sardines
» Salmon with bones
» White beans
» Almonds
» Seaweed

Calcium—the foundation: The current recommendation for calcium intake for the midlife crowd is 1,000 to 1,200 mg every day. The average American consumes about 300 mg per day, so most of us have a lot of catching up to do.

What is the best way of making sure you get enough calcium? This is a subject of much debate in the medical community. For a long time, menopausal women were advised to take calcium supplements for bone health. But some research has suggested that too much calcium through supplementation may put women at a higher risk for heart attack and kidney stones. Although this association remains controversial, it reinforces the recommendation that we should *eat* our daily calcium requirement in food sources rather than rely on supplementation with over-the-counter tablets. Additionally, calcium is best absorbed from food. So your homework assignment is to eat more calcium rich foods. Would someone please pass me the plate of sardines?

If you still find you are not eating sufficient calcium every day, it is absolutely fine to supplement daily with a 500 mg calcium tablet. I prefer Citracal Petites because it is calcium citrate, which absorbs easily without food. It also contains the right amount of vitamin D, and the tablets are indeed petite!

Vitamin D—calcium's "helper": We also need vitamin D to make this bone health strategy work. The job of vitamin D is to help get calcium absorbed into the bloodstream from our intestine. It is also necessary for maintaining adequate calcium levels in our body. Back in our younger days, most of us got vitamin D by sitting in the sun and getting a tan, because vitamin D is made in the skin through solar ultraviolet radiation. Who remembers those 1970s Coppertone commercials?

Unfortunately, as you learned in chapter 9, "Who Is That Wrinkly Old Woman in the Mirror?," that kind of sun exposure is also the best way to get skin damage, wrinkles, and skin cancer. We really do get a lot of ambient sun exposure without needing to lie flat on a towel for hours. However, as we grow older, our skin becomes less efficient at producing vitamin D, even when exposed to the sun. So wear your sunscreen and take vitamin D in the amount of 600 to 1,000 IU every day. You can take a vitamin D tablet alone or in combination with a calcium supplement.

Make sure to get your vitamin D blood level checked every couple of years. If it is between 20 and 50 ng/ml, you are doing a good job. If it is less than that, you will need higher amounts of vitamin D to fill up the tank. If it is higher, you will need to back down. A few years ago, I checked my own level and found it to be significantly low. That's because I avoid the hot summer sun, wear fabulous protective hats, and apply lots of Neutrogena Ultra Sheer Dry-Touch Broad Spectrum SPF 30 on my face, neck, hands, and anywhere else that needs protecting. In order to get my level back to normal, I had to take a prescription strength dose of vitamin D for three months. Now I make sure to take a vitamin D tablet every morning.

By the way, some of you may be taking *too much* vitamin D, because you have been told that it will reduce your risk of cancer, diabetes, and heart and autoimmune disease. This reduction in risk is very controversial. That old saying still rings true—"More is not always better." More is just more, and that may be harmful. So stick with the current recommendations.

STAND TALL AND DON'T FALL DOWN

Perhaps the best preventive measure is to avoid falling. Does that sound both silly and obvious? It turns out that falling down is the number one cause of hip fractures, *the most dreaded bone attack of all*. Vertebral fractures, on the other hand, are usually not caused by falling. They occur silently and are the most common reason we get shorter and hunch over.

Fall Prevention Tips

» Wear sensible shoes.
» Remove clutter.
» Light up the stairway.
» Use nonskid rugs.
» Drink less alcohol.
» Install shower grab bars.
» Avoid walking outside after snowstorms!

DON'T BE A LAZYBONES

Physical activity plays an important role in the prevention of osteoporosis and fracture. Many of us have been doing aerobic exercises for years. Now, however, we have to add in strength training and targeted exercises for fall prevention. The secret here is to add light weights and core balance exercises to our regimen at least several times a week. Tai Chi, anyone? I will cover this in greater detail in chapter 18, "Do I Really Have to Lifts Weights Too?"

I TRIED EVERYTHING AND STILL DEVELOPED OSTEOPOROSIS!

Despite the fact that many of you have already implemented all the necessary lifestyle changes to protect your bones, some of you will still get osteopenia or osteoporosis. Remember that age, genetics, menopausal bone loss, and certain medical conditions and medications are also at play. If you have either osteopenia with additional risk factors or osteoporosis, you will definitely need to take prescription medication. No amount of calcium, vitamin D, and weight training can protect you from a bone attack if you've gotten this far down the line.

There are several FDA-approved medication options for the prevention and treatment of osteoporosis and fracture. One of them is hormone therapy, which I will cover in chapter 16, "Potions, Patches, and Pills, Oh My!" This is a particularly good choice for the younger symptomatic menopause crowd, since you get a lot of bang for your buck with both the treatment of flashes and the protection of bone. There are also some really exciting new therapies being developed for the treatment of osteoporosis that will be able to restore both bone mass and strength. And for those of you who have been listening to the sensationalized news reports about the use of bisphosphonates and the complication of osteonecrosis of the jaw and atypical femur fracture, you should know that the majority of those *rare* cases occur in cancer patients who are taking ten times the doses that you require. So stop worrying about it. But even if you need prescription medication, bone healthy lifestyle changes are still very important. And remember the best advice of all . . . do not fall down! I mean it.

Prescription Drugs for Osteoporosis

» Bisphosphonates
» Hormone therapy
» Zoledronic acid
» Estrogen agonists/antagonists
» Calcitonin
» Parathyroid hormone
» RANK ligand inhibitor

Osteoporosis and broken bones are *not* part of normal aging. There is a lot we can do throughout our lives to keep our bones healthy and walk tall!

CHAPTER 15

I Left My Heart in San Francisco

I am strong. I am invincible. I am woman!

—HELEN REDDY

TRUST ME WHEN I tell you that I do not love being the bearer of disheartening news. However, I cannot tiptoe around the fact that heart disease is the leading cause of death in American women. Astonishingly, more than 400,000 women will die every year from this disease. It is a staggering number, and higher than the number of deaths annually from cancer, Alzheimer's, lung disease, and accidents *combined*. One out of three women will die from heart disease, which works out to be about one death per minute. Tick tock on my clock.

Even still, most of us don't truly appreciate the gravity of the situation. So how about this statistic to get your attention? The lifetime risk for heart disease is high in almost *all* women, approaching an incredible one out of two. So it turns out, Helen Reddy, that when it comes to heart disease, women are not invincible after all. I really do love your song, though. Much to the husband's dismay, I sing "I Am Woman" all the time.

The purpose of this chapter is to raise awareness and to focus your attention on the prevention of heart disease, a term that I will use broadly to include a bunch of medical issues like high blood pressure, heart attack, stroke, and blood clots.

So what can women do about all this bad news? Well, why don't we do what we always do? When someone hands us a lemon, it's time to roll up our sleeves and make some delicious lemonade. Only now, as you will soon learn, we will have to add a lot less sugar. Luckily, girls are already made of sugar and spice and everything nice.

EQUAL RIGHTS AT LAST

The menopausal transition is a particularly important time of life to take stock of your risk of heart disease, because risk increases as estrogen levels decrease. This is especially true for younger women who go through early menopause either from surgery to remove their ovaries or because of a variety of other medical conditions. When it comes to getting a heart attack, menopausal women of every age finally begin to achieve equal rights with men! I am quite sure this was not one of the goals that Gloria Steinem had in mind at the start of the women's movement back in the 1960s.

ARE THERE ANY RISK TAKERS AMONG US?

I will let you in on a little secret. I am not a risk taker. When I'm in Las Vegas, I skip the gambling tables and head right for a show. I loved seeing Celine Dion recently, and I am looking forward to checking out J. Lo the next time I'm in Sin City. When it comes to heart health, we all need to play it safe. So let's start doing absolutely everything we can to avoid being a statistic.

The American Heart Association (AHA) has issued a set of guidelines for heart disease prevention. Risk is divided into three categories. The goal is to be in the *"ideal risk"* group. If you fall into either the *"at risk"* or *"high risk"* group, bless your heart, you will need to consult a cardiologist.

Ideal Risk

All of the following:

» Total cholesterol <200 mg/dL
» Blood pressure <120/80 mm Hg
» Fasting blood sugar <100 mg/dL
» BMI <25 kg/m2
» Healthy diet
» No cigarette smoking
» Moderate intensity physical activity ≥150 minutes/ week
   or
» Vigorous intensity exercise ≥75 minutes/week

To be considered ideal risk, you cannot be taking medication to achieve any of the targets above. You have to get there all by yourself!

At Risk

One or more of the following:

» Total cholesterol ≥200 mg/dL
» HDL cholesterol <50 mg/dL
» Systolic blood pressure ≥120 mm Hg
» Diastolic blood pressure ≥80 mm Hg
» High blood pressure treated with medication
» Abnormal cholesterol treated with medication
» High blood pressure or diabetes during pregnancy

» Metabolic syndrome
» Autoimmune collagen vascular disease *(e.g., lupus or rheumatoid arthritis)*
» Family history of premature heart disease in first degree relatives *(men <55 years old or women <65 years old)*
» Poor diet
» Cigarette smoking
» Physical inactivity
» Obesity
» Central belly fat

High Risk

One or more of the following:

» Established heart disease
» Peripheral vascular disease
» Diabetes
» Cerebrovascular disease

» Chronic kidney disease
» Abdominal aortic aneurism
» 10-year predicted heart disease risk of ≥10%

Your 10-year risk assessment calculation includes:

» Gender
» Age
» Race
» Cholesterol levels

» Blood pressure
» Diabetes
» Cigarette smoking status

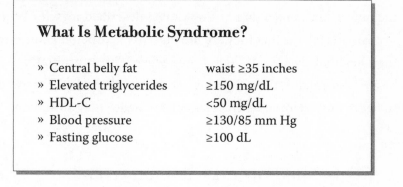

What Is Metabolic Syndrome?

» Central belly fat   waist ≥35 inches
» Elevated triglycerides   ≥150 mg/dL
» HDL-C   <50 mg/dL
» Blood pressure   ≥130/85 mm Hg
» Fasting glucose   ≥100 dL

NO TIME LEFT FOR EXCUSES

As most midlife women already know, if you are experiencing perimenopausal or menopausal symptoms, you are less likely to have the energy and stamina necessary to exercise daily and eat healthily. So if you are too tired and cranky because you have been flashing and sweating all night . . . well, that's a horse of a different color. As you will learn in chapter 16, "Potions, Patches, and Pills, Oh My!," *some* of you will not be able to make much headway into your new and improved healthy lifestyle choices until you've gotten a handle on your symptoms. Believe me when I say that I completely understand. You may even want to skip ahead to chapter 17, "I Want to Feel like a Natural Woman," for the latest information on non-hormonal approaches to symptom relief. Once you start feeling better, please return to this section to resume learning about how to lower your risk of heart disease.

By the way, there is a whole category of women out there who have not yet gotten on the healthy lifestyle bandwagon. You know who you are. I refer to this group as the "Too Busy Bodies." I get it. You are just too busy. I take care of a lot of Too Busy Bodies who have demanding jobs, a husband who does not help enough around the house, kids, and a dog. (I think I just described myself.) When my patients tell me that they are too busy to make better choices for their health, I always ask, "If not now, when?" That turns out not to be a rhetorical question. Together, we review every day of the week to figure out where small changes can be made. They all add up.

AHA! THE EXERCISE GUIDELINES

Believe it or not, there are actual heart health exercise guidelines that we should all be following to reduce our risk of heart disease. When midlife women exercise regularly, we are able to maintain a lower weight, blood pressure, and blood sugar levels.

The AHA recommends that women get *at least* 150 minutes per week of moderate intensity aerobic exercise like brisk walking or 75 minutes per week of vigorous exercise like a high energy cycle class.

I just shoveled snow for 15 minutes, which really got my heart rate up and definitely counts toward my weekly requirement. When I lived in San Francisco, I used to take a salsa dance class. It was both sexy and sweaty! I will reveal my own exercise regimen in chapter 18, "Do I Really Have to Lift Weights Too?" There is just no end to the variety of aerobic activities we can enjoy as we focus on the goal of heart health.

AHA! THE DIETARY GUIDELINES

As you'll recall, there are new *general* dietary guidelines that I reviewed in chapter 7, "What's the Skinny on Weight Gain?" Below,

I have summarized the specific American Heart Association recommendations for the prevention of heart disease.

Fruits and vegetables	≥4.5 cups/day
Fish	Twice/week
Fiber	30 gm/day
Whole grains	3 servings/day
Sugar	Just a spoonful 5 times/ week
Nuts, legumes, and seeds	4 servings/week
Saturated fats	Reduce fried foods, dessert, butter, and cheese
Cholesterol	Reduce meat and eggs
Sodium	1,500 mg/day
Alcohol	≤1/day (4 oz. wine or 12 oz. beer or 1.5 oz. 80-proof spirits)

I'LL HAVE A MARTINI, STRAIGHT UP

According to the American Heart Association, there is scientific
research demonstrating that drinking alcohol in moderation is
associated with a decreased risk of heart disease. The mechanism
for this has to do with alcohol's effect on increasing HDL, the good

component of cholesterol. Alcohol may also have some antioxidant and anticlotting properties, which turn out to be good for heart health too.

And despite the fact that red wine seems to get all the credit, any alcohol will do the job. So whether you enjoy beer, chardonnay, a mint julep, or moonshine, you can continue to do so . . . in moderation. That means only one glass per day at most. And if you do not drink alcohol, this is not an invitation to start. There are better ways to protect your heart, like lowering bad cholesterol, controlling high blood pressure, eating a healthy diet, getting physically fit, and maintaining a normal weight. Having said that, I am always just a tad more relaxed and even a little bit giggly after I've enjoyed a Bombay Sapphire gin martini with a lemon twist.

There are, of course, risks related to drinking too much alcohol including alcoholism, high blood pressure, obesity, stroke, breast cancer, suicide, and accidents. I don't mean to spoil the party. Please drink responsibly or not at all.

SHOULD WOMEN TAKE A DAILY LOW-DOSE ASPIRIN?

Before scientific studies on heart health were designed to focus specifically on women, the recommendations we were told to follow reflected the information gathered on men. While many heart health recommendations for both women and men are still the same, the use of aspirin took a decidedly sharp left turn when applied to primary prevention of heart attacks in women. As it turns out, while low-dose aspirin has been routinely recommended for the primary prevention of heart attacks in men, the story for women is more complicated.

In 2005, the Women's Health Study (WHS) was the first and largest trial designed to study the benefits and risks of low-dose aspirin use in women to *prevent* heart attacks and stroke. The results showed that for most healthy women who were less than sixty-five years old, routine use of aspirin was *not recommended* for the primary prevention of heart attacks or stroke, because the risks of bleeding in the gastrointestinal tract and brain outweighed the benefits. For women who were sixty-five and older, the WHS showed that low-dose aspirin was beneficial for the *primary* prevention of heart attacks and stroke. However, no formal recommendations were established because no one seemed to agree on who should take a daily low-dose aspirin.

To make the muddy waters even muddier, new guidelines released by the USPSTF lump men and women together. They recommend the use of low-dose aspirin for primary prevention of heart attacks and stroke in the fifty- to fifty-nine-year-old group if you have a 10 percent or greater ten year heart disease risk and expect to live for at least ten more years. As you have already learned in chapter 12, "Hooray for Colonoscopy!" the use of aspirin in this age group can reduce the risk of colon cancer too. The catch is that you must commit to taking daily low-dose aspirin for the full ten years in order to benefit. The USPSTF recommendations for the over-sixty crowd get more complicated and require someone with an MD, PhD, and Nobel Prize to decipher.

So I will leave you with my best advice on this important and complicated question. No matter what age you are, the best strategy for the prevention of heart disease in women is to follow the AHA exercise and dietary guidelines. As for whether or not you should consider taking a low-dose aspirin for the primary prevention of heart attack, stroke, and colon cancer, please walk briskly to your nearest healthcare professional or cardiologist for the best individu-alized approach. Hopefully, they are toting around the new aspirin-guide decision support tool available on most mobile devices to help figure it all out.

DOES ESTROGEN THERAPY PREVENT HEART DISEASE?

The pendulum has swung back and forth so many times on this issue over the past few decades that if you are not careful, you might get hit in the head. And if I don't explain everything very carefully now, I am certain that one of my colleagues will be tempted to hit me over the head with my own book. So let's all take a deep breath and learn about how estrogen can be both helpful as well as harmful to the heart.

There have been plenty of scientific studies that have demon-strated estrogen therapy's protective role in heart health. The mecha-nism for this positive association is complicated and has to do with the fact that estrogen inhibits the development of atherosclerosis, increases good HDL cholesterol, lowers bad LDL cholesterol, keeps blood sugar levels under control, relaxes blood vessels, and helps maintain normal arterial blood flow.

Simultaneously, however, estrogen therapy can also harm the heart, because it can increase triglycerides, which contribute to the development of atherosclerosis. Estrogen therapy also promotes clotting and inflammation inside blood vessels, which can lead to heart attacks, stroke, deep venous thrombosis, and pulmonary embolism. When women hear only this part of the story, they usu-ally start running for the hills. Well, at least that counts toward our weekly exercise requirement. You can read the complete story on risks and benefits of hormone therapy in the next chapter, "Potions, Patches, and Pills, Oh My!," but I will give you the estrogen-heart story here.

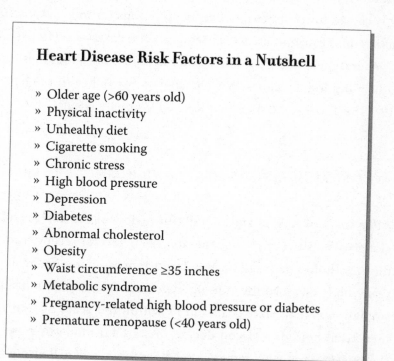

Heart Disease Risk Factors in a Nutshell

» Older age (>60 years old)
» Physical inactivity
» Unhealthy diet
» Cigarette smoking
» Chronic stress
» High blood pressure
» Depression
» Diabetes
» Abnormal cholesterol
» Obesity
» Waist circumference ≥35 inches
» Metabolic syndrome
» Pregnancy-related high blood pressure or diabetes
» Premature menopause (<40 years old)

For decades, women were encouraged to use estrogen therapy specifically to prevent heart disease. This recommendation was based, in part, on results from the 1976 Nurses' Health Study (NHS). Fast-forward to the late 1980s, where data from the Postmenopausal Estrogen/Progestin Interventions (PEPI) trial showed that the use of estrogen therapy could reduce heart disease by 30 percent. However, in the 1990s, a very large, complex, and expensive study called the Women's Health Initiative (WHI) was designed to really get to the heart of the matter. When the study results started to trickle out in 2002, an avalanche of terror followed. The healthcare community was blindsided and confused. The media immediately sensationalized and misrepresented the story. And the initial WHI message to women, that hormone therapy causes heart attacks, stroke, deep venous thrombosis, pulmonary embolism, and breast cancer, has left a devastating impact on a generation of midlife women. You can read more about these and other important studies that changed women's health in chapter 19, "The Top Five Studies That Rocked Women's Health."

THE BOTTOM LINE ON HEART AND HORMONE THERAPY

After years of careful and thoughtful review of the WHI results, along with critical new information from several recent studies, the take-home message on this important women's health issue really boils down to the "timing hypothesis." If you are a healthy woman, less than sixty years old or within ten years of your last menstrual period, and you decide to start hormone therapy for the treatment of your menopausal symptoms, you will also enjoy the benefits of improved heart health and a decrease in your total mortality risk. This is especially true if you went through early menopause or had a hysterectomy, and therefore do not need to take progesterone, as you will learn in the next chapter, "Potions, Patches, and Pills, Oh My!"

On the other hand, if you have waited more than ten years from your last menstrual period or have reached your midsixties before considering hormone therapy, it is too late. Elvis has left the building. The risks are now greater than the benefits. The secret is to start hormone therapy early, when your heart is young and healthy.

WHAT I KNOW FOR SURE . . . AS OPRAH WOULD SAY!

It would be *ideal* if all women would strive to achieve ideal risk status when it comes to preventing heart disease. If only we, as younger twenty-somethings, took heart health seriously, we wouldn't be facing such a deep fried pickle at midlife. As Momma used to say, "Too soon old, too late smart." However, it is not too late. To quote the poet Maya Angelou, "I did then what I knew how to do. Now that I know better, I do better."

CHAPTER 16

Potions, Patches, and Pills, Oh My!

There is no more creative force in the world
than the menopausal woman with zest.

—MARGARET MEAD

HORMONE THERAPY DECISIONS ARE scary for many women. It is just like when Dorothy, the Scarecrow, the Tin Man, and the Cowardly Lion go deep into the forest on an adventure to find the Wizard of Oz, someone they hope can help them with solutions to their problems. Along the way, they are terrified of encountering lions, tigers, and bears, oh my! Well, it is just the same for you. As you head off on your own journey to discover the mysteries of hormone therapy, a term that is used to describe estrogen, progesterone, and testosterone treatments available to menopausal women, you are faced with all kinds of conflicting and sometimes wrong information in newspapers and magazines and on TV and the Internet. Even your trusted healthcare professional may give you incorrect advice. I see this all the time. As it turns out, not every gynecologist knows everything in the rapidly changing landscape of hormone therapy.

So how are you supposed to know if hormone therapy is the right choice for you? Which is the best one? What if you try something and it doesn't work? Who can help you find your way? Well, I can, of course. By the end of this chapter, you will understand all the who, what, when, why, and how of hormone therapy. Knowledge is power. So get ready to become empowered!

ANOTHER HISTORY LESSON

The word *menopause* was derived from the Greek words *men* and *pausis*, meaning the cessation of menstrual cycles. Now you finally know how the word *men* nestled itself into an entire branch of women's health. As you will read in chapter 20, "Every Man Needs a Gynecologist," the menfolk really do play an important role.

Thousands of years ago, Aristotle wrote about the connection between the end of menstruation and a woman's fertility. Fast-forward to a letter written in the 1800s by American obstetrician Charles Meigs titled "Change of Life" where he asks, "What has she to expect, save grey hairs, wrinkles and the gradual decay of these physical and personal attractions?" Thanks a lot, Charlie!

By the late 1800s, however, the scientific community in Europe introduced the modern concept of hormone therapy for the treatment of menopause symptoms. And by the mid-1900s, women were being routinely offered estrogen so they could stay young, beautiful, and "Feminine Forever." Once it was determined that women with a uterus also needed progesterone to avoid getting uterine cancer, that got thrown into the mix too.

It was not until the 1970s that better scientific studies focusing on midlife women were designed. Until then, most recommendations for women's health were derived from studies done on men. And as we all know, women are not men. A funny patient of mine once told me that the problem with men is that they are not women! That sounds like a good title for my next book. By the way, I hope that all of you science geeks out there will enjoy chapter 19, "The Top Five Studies That Rocked Women's Health."

PERIMENOPAUSE IS NOT MENOPAUSE

As you'll recall from chapter 3, "My Husband Thinks I'm Crazy," the physiology of perimenopause is different from that of menopause. Perimenopausal women are usually in their forties and still making estrogen and progesterone from their hardworking but aging ovaries. However, that production is erratic and unpredictable. Menopausal women, on the other hand, are all done with the job of making estrogen and progesterone from their ovaries. As for the production of testosterone, that continues for both groups until a few years beyond the last menstrual period. And then, ladies, we are out of testosterone too.

PERIMENOPAUSAL SYMPTOM RELIEF

For those in the Perimenopause Club, you are not yet candidates for hormone therapy. I know you are suffering mightily with hot flashes, night sweats, sleep problems, mood issues, brain fog, reduced libido, and so much more. Just think of yourselves as *too young* for hormone therapy! Yep, that's right. You are not menopausal yet, and you will have to patiently wait your turn. That is terrific news, though, because you will not have to get into a long, complicated, and confusing discussion about the risks of hormone therapy. That day will come eventually.

So what is the best treatment option for the symptomatic perimenopausal woman? I would now like a drumroll, please. It turns out that the *continuous use of a low-dose birth control pill,* which is a combination of a synthetic estrogen and progesterone, is the right choice for women in their forties and early fifties who still have ovarian function. The goal is to get off your hormonal roller-coaster ride and onto the easy tram ride. Ironically, the hormone doses in birth control pills are much higher than those of hormone therapy. That is necessary in order for the pills to take over the reins from your wild and crazy ovaries.

Did anyone notice that I emphasized the word *continuous*? Here comes a new concept. When birth control pills are used in younger women, a pill break is typically built into the monthly prescription. That allows women to have an artificial withdrawal bleed that feels like a period. There is absolutely no scientific reason to do it this way. Just as in that song from *Fiddler on the Roof,* it is "Tradition!"

For the symptomatic perimenopausal crowd, it is much better to take a low-dose birth control pill every single day of the week, month, and year without a break. I know that this will be shocking to many of you. Why hasn't anyone told you this before? Is it really safe? Shouldn't we give our bodies a rest from pills every once in a while? Don't we need to shed the uterine lining for health reasons?

Nope, we do not. Over time, with continuous exposure to low-dose birth control pills, the lining of the uterus will flatten out. There may be some unscheduled spotting and bleeding for a few months along the way, but most uterine linings will get the hang of this new-and-improved program within about a year. The whole idea behind this strategy is to give your unreliable ovaries a vacation

Benefits of Birth Control Pills (Big)

» Contraception
» Decreased or no bleeding
» Money saved on tampons, pads, and ibuprofen
» PMS relief
» Acne improvement
» Perimenopause symptoms relief
» Fewer biopsies for benign breast disease
» Ovarian and uterine cancer risk reduction

Nuisances of Birth Control Pills (Medium)

» Nausea
» Headache
» Bloating
» Breast tenderness
» Reduced libido
» Spotting or bleeding

Risks of Birth Control Pills (Small)

» Blood clots
» Heart attack
» Stroke

while simultaneously supplying your brain with a reliable daily dose of estrogen. If you were to take a break from low-dose birth control pills, your symptoms would just return full throttle. Roller coasters, start your engines. The bitch is back!

You Cannot Take Birth Control Pills If You Have Had . . .

» A blood clot
» A pulmonary embolism
» A heart attack
» A stroke
» Untreated high blood pressure
» Severe diabetes
» Or are a cigarette smoker over the age of 35

THE BIG DECISION (AT LEAST FOR NOW)

Which low-dose birth control pill is the best one of all? I am fond of telling my patients that they make many different kinds of birth control pills, because they make many different kinds of women. All birth control pills contain the same synthetic estrogen, ethinyl estradiol. However, the dose of estrogen and the type of synthetic progesterone will differ.

I always start my perimenopausal patients off with a 20 mcg dose pill. When it comes to the synthetic progesterone component, there are some subtle differences that I factor into my decision making process. I tailor my choices based on patient history and insurance coverage. No need to spend more when you can spend less. And this brings me right back to my earlier advice, which is to find a healthcare professional who is very knowledgeable about perimenopause and menopause. Otherwise, you will spin your wheels and get nowhere fast.

For all of you perimenopausal girls who are not candidates for low-dose birth control pills, your healthcare professional will have to individualize your treatment choices based on your specific situation.

By the way, there are no "bioidentical" birth control pills. That term applies only to a particular hormone therapy. And most important, if you are a smoker over the age of thirty-five, you cannot take birth control pills. So quit smoking, for crying out loud. Or your perimenopausal symptoms will keep you crying out loud!

PERIMENOPAUSE TREATMENT WRAP-UP

Here is how the perimenopause journey ends. Those of you who are candidates for a continuous low-dose birth control pill should start right away, regardless of where you are in your cycle. You do not need to wait for the traditional Sunday start day. The sooner you take your low-dose pills, the sooner you will get symptom relief. I always recommend taking them at bedtime. That way, if you have any nuisance side effects, you will be sound asleep and not notice. Expect to feel relief from your symptoms after about three months of continuous pill use. If you are lucky, you might feel better much sooner. Don't quit the program before the three-month mark, though. That is a mistake a lot of women make. You have to be in it to win it. If you are still experiencing mood symptoms like depression after that time frame, you should consider adding in an antidepressant or anxiety medicine, because your mood symptoms may really be due to an actual depression or anxiety syndrome. If you are experiencing annoying breakthrough bleeding or spotting during the first year of this regimen, be reassured that most nuisance side effects resolve on their own within a few months. You can nip this bleeding issue in the blooming bud by wearing an estrogen patch for one or two weeks, which stabilizes the lining of the uterus. If you're still experiencing unscheduled bleeding after a year, it's time to have a looky-loo inside your uterus with a pelvic ultrasound.

How long should perimenopausal women take continuous low-dose birth control pills for symptom relief? It is generally recommended that you stick with them until the age of fifty-five. By then, most women will have transitioned through menopause and will land more comfortably on the other side of debilitating symptoms. By doing it this way, you will never officially know when your last menstrual period occurred, because being on the pill stops natural cycles. But don't spend one minute fretting about this fact. The benefits of perimenopausal symptom relief far outweigh a proper farewell to your last ovulated egg.

By the way, there are always a few fifty-five-year-old holdouts who are not yet menopausal and still have some old eggs left to ovulate. Show-offs! If that turns out to be you, the solution is to go back on your low-dose birth control pill for another year. If at first you don't succeed, try, try again. Most women love their continuous regimen, because it works well, is easy to use, and has no controversy involved. It is always a bittersweet moment when I have to graduate a patient from the Perimenopause Club and admit them into the Menopause Club. That is when the decisions get more challenging.

Once you are considered menopausal, the decision to use hormone therapy will depend on the severity of your symptoms, personal preferences, medical and family history, and whether you have found the right healthcare professional to guide you properly.

THE SECRETS OF HORMONE THERAPY REVEALED

There are 65 million menopausal women in the United States, and most of you are not using hormone therapy. I think that's because so many of you are either too terrified of the risks or have no idea where to start. Well, it's always best to start at the beginning.

The most important decision you can make for yourself at this stage of life is to invest in your own health and wellness. There is no time left to procrastinate. I know that you have heard this many times before. But, gosh darn it, you need to hear it again. Menopause shines a white-hot light on a terrific opportunity to take stock of your lifestyle choices and improve in all areas. Now is the time for daily exercise, good nutrition, a healthy body weight, stress reduction, and avoiding cigarette smoking.

Here comes the catch-22. It is practically impossible to gear up for Yin Yoga when you feel lousy and tired. So which does indeed come first—the chicken or the egg? I've always wanted to answer this question. I'll say "Chicken." In fact, you may need to start a treatment regimen *first* to give you the get-up-and-go to get up and go!

As you will read in chapter 17, "I Want to Feel like a Natural Woman," you can begin your menopause symptom relief journey by trying nonhormonal options. So if you want to skip to that chapter now, I will wait for you. For those of you who are ready to take the trip into the wonderful world of hormone therapy, follow me.

SYSTEMIC ESTROGEN THERAPY

Estrogen therapy is the *most effective* treatment for hot flashes, night sweats, and vaginal dryness. You will need to take estrogen *systemically* to relieve most menopausal symptoms. This means that the estrogen will be absorbed into your bloodstream and travel everywhere from your head to your toe and all the areas in between. The exception to that rule is the use of *local* estrogen used specifically for the treatment of vaginal dryness, painful sex, and the prevention of recurrent bladder infections. More on that in a moment.

Systemic estrogen therapy comes in the forms of a pill, patch, spray, gel, and vaginal ring. The delivery system choices are generally divided into oral (a pill) versus transdermal (everything else). Most of you will be able to have all of the choices at your disposal. The reasons to consider one approach over another will be based on your personal preference regarding taking a daily pill, wearing a patch once or twice a week, slathering a gel on different parts of your body, or sticking a silicone ring into your vagina every three months. I know the last choice sounds off-putting, but it works great for so many women who don't want to be bothered with a daily or weekly regimen. Your healthcare professional may also have some strong opinions based on clinical experience and your personal medical history.

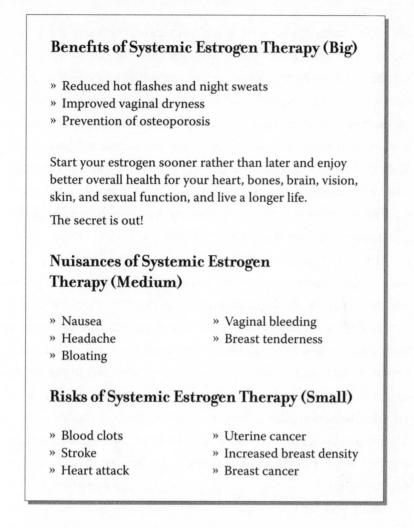

Benefits of Systemic Estrogen Therapy (Big)

» Reduced hot flashes and night sweats
» Improved vaginal dryness
» Prevention of osteoporosis

Start your estrogen sooner rather than later and enjoy better overall health for your heart, bones, brain, vision, skin, and sexual function, and live a longer life.

The secret is out!

Nuisances of Systemic Estrogen Therapy (Medium)

» Nausea
» Headache
» Bloating
» Vaginal bleeding
» Breast tenderness

Risks of Systemic Estrogen Therapy (Small)

» Blood clots
» Stroke
» Heart attack
» Uterine cancer
» Increased breast density
» Breast cancer

AGE MATTERS, AND TIMING IS EVERYTHING
(TWO CLICHÉS FOR THE PRICE OF ONE!)

Here is how I manage my own patients, which is based on all of the available scientific studies. If you fall into the fifty- to fifty-nine-year-old age group, I consider you my *youngsters*. If you are younger than that, I suppose you are my pre-youngsters. When it comes to taking hormone therapy, all of you youngsters out there are at very low risk because of your youth. And for those of you who have put off the decision to try hormone therapy while you either tough it out or use other approaches, if you are within ten years of your last menstrual period, you are still a candidate for estrogen therapy. If you are more than ten years from your last menstrual period, you are out of luck. You have missed your opportunity. At this point, the risks will outweigh the benefits. But don't be glum. As luck would have it, the very next chapter, "I Want to Feel like a Natural Woman," covers plenty of nonhormonal solutions.

How do I guide your choices? Unless you have any specific personal or medical issues that might lead me in a particular direction, you get to try any of the available therapies that resonate with you. I choose the dose based on the severity of your symptoms, extenuating medical conditions, and your personal preference. If you have no strong feelings one way or the other, I usually start in the middle dose range, so there is room to go up or down as needed. Then we stick to this regimen for three months, unless there is a darn tootin' good reason to change it sooner. If our first approach is not working after three months, we adjust the dose or delivery system accordingly.

Once you hit your sixties, I strongly recommend using lower doses as well as a transdermal approach, because the risk profile is slightly better. I almost never recommend that women stop estrogen therapy altogether, unless a medical reason intervenes. The North American Menopause Society recently issued a statement on continuing use of systemic hormone therapy after the age of sixty-five. In a nutshell, when estrogen is started within ten years of your last menstrual period, it plays a very important and positive role in preserving heart, bone, brain, sexual, and overall health and wellness.

This is no longer controversial. It just takes a while for everyone to hear the medical message. And even though the risks from taking *any* medication increase as we age, there is no reason that the sixty- and seventy-somethings should not continue to enjoy overall health and wellness too.

You Cannot Take Systemic Estrogen Therapy If You Have:

» Unexplained vaginal bleeding
» Liver disease
» Gallbladder disease
» Blood-clotting disorder
» Pulmonary embolism
» Untreated high blood pressure
» Heart attack
» Uterine cancer
» Breast cancer

THE ELEPHANT IN THE ROOM JOINS THE LIONS, TIGERS, AND BEARS, OH MY!

For most you, the fear of breast cancer turns out to be the most common reason you avoid or discontinue systemic estrogen therapy. Fear is always the elephant in the room. The reality is that systemic estrogen therapy, used for longer than seven years, has been associated with a *very small* increase in breast cancer. However, systemic estrogen therapy does not cause your normal breast cell to become cancerous. The mechanism for this increase is due to the fact that systemic estrogen can help a tiny breast cancer cell that you already have hiding in your breast, not yet seen on mammogram, grow up. The chance of this happening takes many years and is really very, very small. You have a better chance of getting eaten by a great big whale.

So unless you said "Yes" to any of the listed reasons in my "You Cannot Take Systemic Estrogen Therapy" box, I don't want fear to stand in your way of improved health. As you learned in chapter 15, "I Left My Heart in San Francisco," the number one killer of women in the United States by a long shot is heart disease. Since systemic estrogen therapy plays a significant role in the protection of heart health when used early in the menopause transition, it is actually more likely to help rather than harm you.

THE BRCA PATIENT

For those who carry the BRCA gene mutation, your journey will be more challenging when it comes to dealing with menopause symptoms. Please review the section "BRCA Gene Testing" (page 117) devoted to you in chapter 11, "It's All About the Breast." Many of you will choose to undergo the removal of your ovaries and fallopian tubes in order to reduce your ovarian cancer risk. Once you become surgically menopausal, your symptoms are more likely to be severe.

So can you try hormone therapy? The answer is absolutely "Yes!" Even though your BRCA status puts you at increased risk for breast cancer too, the addition of systemic hormone therapy to treat your severe symptoms will not increase your baseline risk any further. And if, at some point, you choose to have your breasts removed to further decrease your breast cancer risk, then your breast cancer worries are over.

LOCAL VAGINAL ESTROGEN THERAPY

For those of you suffering from vaginal dryness, painful inter-course, or recurrent bladder infections, you don't need to look any further than local vaginal estrogen therapy. The advantage of treating your specific vaginal and bladder symptoms locally means that you will not have to worry about the risks attributed to sys-temic estrogen therapy. As mentioned, the FDA requires that all estrogen products contain the same warnings. Don't be fright-ened by what you read on the package label when it comes to local estrogen therapy.

Your choices include a twice-weekly vaginal tablet or cream or a silicone ring inserted into the vagina every three months. I should mention that some of you may need to use your local estrogen ther-apy more frequently than just twice a week. If you are not feeling enough improvement of your vaginal dryness after three months, increase your interval to three times per week for another few months. In fact, I have some patients who use their local estrogen therapy every night, because that is what works best for them. It will take time to figure out what works best for you.

How long should you use local vaginal estrogen therapy? I always say, "*Forever,* or until you no longer want a healthy vagina." Remember, when it comes to local estrogen therapy, what goes in the vagina, stays in the vagina! Feel free to review chapter 6, "The Vagina Is like Las Vegas, *Baby!*"

Finally, there is a new kid on the block called ospemifene, which is the only FDA-approved nonestrogen treatment for painful sex caused by vaginal dryness in menopause. It falls in the class of selec-tive estrogen receptor modulator (SERM). Because it is a daily pill taken by mouth, I recommend this choice to women who do not like to fuss with their vaginas.

PROGESTERONE THERAPY

Progesterone has only one job when it comes to symptomatic menopausal women. If you are taking estrogen and you have a uterus, progesterone is added to protect your uterus from the stimulating effects of estrogen on the uterine lining. If you took only estrogen, you would put your uterus at risk for an abnormal condition known as hyperplasia and uterine cancer. So if you have had a hysterectomy, and therefore do not have a uterus, you *do not* need to take progesterone. Case closed.

For those of you who have a uterus, what is your best progesterone choice? There are several preparations available, but I am going to reveal my favorite one. I strongly prefer the micronized progesterone pill taken every night at bedtime or cycled for fourteen nights, either monthly or every three months. Based on all of the available scientific information and my own clinical experience, it appears to be the safest and most well tolerated.

For those of you who cannot tolerate a progesterone pill, your next best choice is a progesterone-containing IUD. This approach works very well, even though it is considered *off label*. That means that the idea to use an IUD in this manner came along later, after the FDA approved it for contraception only. Don't let that concept confuse you. We use many medications off label. It is a perfectly acceptable thing to do. A good example of this is the off-label use of low-dose birth control pills for anything besides contraception. Please review the "Benefits of Birth Control Pills" box. By the way, we really must stop bad-mouthing IUDs. They are the most effective reversible contraception available, and their reputation continues to suffer because of one bad apple, the Dalkon Shield, which has not been around for decades.

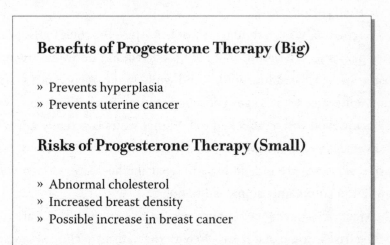

Benefits of Progesterone Therapy (Big)

» Prevents hyperplasia
» Prevents uterine cancer

Risks of Progesterone Therapy (Small)

» Abnormal cholesterol
» Increased breast density
» Possible increase in breast cancer

There is another new kid on the block called DUAVEE that is an FDA-approved combination hormone therapy with both estrogen and a SERM. This is another good choice for women who cannot tolerate progesterone.

As for the use of progesterone cream or gel for the protection of the uterus, it is absolutely not recommended, because it has not been scientifically proven to work consistently. Do not put your uterus at risk for hyperplasia or cancer. Another case closed.

TESTOSTERONE THERAPY

The reason women consider testosterone therapy is specifically for the symptom of low libido, a very common perimenopause and menopause complaint. The difference between these two groups is that perimenopausal women are still making plenty of testosterone, so they will not benefit from any more. Menopausal women, too, continue to make testosterone for about five years beyond their last menstrual period.

Surprisingly, even though one of testosterone's roles in the body is to get us in the mood, there is no correlation between low testosterone levels and low libido. And while many of you with sexual function issues want to get your testosterone levels checked to see if it is low, you will be shocked to find that yours is actually normal. Conversely, you may have a normal libido and find out that your testosterone levels are indeed low. So what the heck are women with low libido complaints supposed to do?

Most of us have lots of good reasons to explain why we are not feeling frisky. Some of it has to do with the natural decline of our sex hormones, but most of it probably does not. So when it comes to considering the use of testosterone therapy for the treatment of low libido, make sure that you have explored absolutely every other reason known to womankind. And then, find a healthcare professional

Risks of Testosterone Therapy (Small to Medium)

» Acne
» Male-pattern hair growth or hair loss
» Deepening voice
» Clitoral enlargement
» Liver dysfunction
» Abnormal cholesterol
» Breast cancer

who *specializes* in sexual health. I do offer women testosterone therapy after very careful consideration. In my experience, testosterone therapy can be helpful for a small segment of the menopause population. However, you should be aware that the FDA has not approved the use of testosterone in women.

Flibanserin is a relatively new medication that is FDA-approved for the treatment of hypoactive sexual desire disorder (HSDD) in *pre*menopausal women. Use in menopausal women is considered off label.

Don't Waste Your Time and Money

Salivary hormone levels are meaningless.

Hormone levels are not helpful if you are on low-dose birth control pills or hormone therapy.

BIOIDENTICAL HORMONE THERAPY

Bioidentical hormones, which include estrogen, progesterone, and testosterone, are often misrepresented as "natural" because they are chemically identical to the hormones that women make in their ovaries. However, bioidentical hormones are definitely not natural. I know that some of you are having trouble believing me, so let me explain it further.

Remember that scene from *I Love Lucy* where Ethel and Lucy are in a big tub, stomping on grapes to make wine? I know that many of you imagine there is some unidentified person mashing up wild yams in a back room to make bioidentical hormones. The reality is that *all* hormone therapy is synthesized in a laboratory.

There are two FDA-approved bioidentical hormone therapy treatment options. The first is *estradiol*, which is available in a pill, patch, lotion, mist, vaginal ring, cream, and tablet. The second is *micronized progesterone*, available in a pill or vaginal gel. There is no scientific data supporting the use of estriol, an estrogen that is made only during pregnancy. The FDA has clearly stated that women should not use bioidentical estriol at all.

Now here comes a very important point. It is much safer to try FDA-approved bioidentical hormone therapy options, because they have undergone rigorous testing for purity, potency, safety, and effectiveness. You should avoid using bioidentical hormone therapy preparations that have been produced in a custom-compounding pharmacy, because they do not undergo any testing whatsoever. It's like the Wild West out there.

THE SUZANNE SOMERS EFFECT

As many of you know, the actress Suzanne Somers has written several books promoting the use of custom-compounded bioidentical hormone therapy for the treatment of menopausal symptoms. She has made the claim that bioidentical hormone therapy is more natural and, therefore, safer. Sometimes, just for fun, I will even refer to her as Dr. Suzanne Somers. Don't get me wrong. I loved the show *Three's Company*. Suzanne is hilarious. You have to be really smart to play dumb. However, Suzanne Somers is not a medical authority on bioidentical hormone therapy. Since you now know that all hormones are synthesized, you will no longer be fooled by claims that lull you into a false sense of security. The bottom line is that all systemic hormone therapy, bioidentical or otherwise, carries the same risk. And unless you are a great horseback-riding sharp shooter, stay out of the custom-compounded Wild West.

NONHORMONAL PRESCRIPTION THERAPY

For those of you who cannot or will not try hormone therapy to treat hot flashes and night sweats, your choices include selective serotonin reuptake inhibitors (SSRIs), serotonin-norepinephrine reuptake inhibitors (SNRIs), and the medications gabapentin and clonidine. In my experience, the SSRIs and SNRIs, which are antidepressants, work the best with the least risk and nuisance side effects. My preferred choices in this group are either the only FDA-approved SSRI for the treatment of hot flashes, which is a low-dose paroxetine mesylate at 7.5 mg, or the SNRI venlafaxine at 37.5 to 75 mg/day. Gabapentin, an antiseizure medication, and clonidine, used to treat high blood pressure, are also effective in treating hot flashes. I tend to avoid using them because they can cause significant side effects that sound a little like the seven dwarfs: Dizzy, Drowsy, Diarrhea, Dry Mouth, Headache, Constipation, and Weight Gain.

SO LITTLE TIME, SO MANY CHOICES

Herein lies the fundamental problem for most healthcare professionals and their symptomatic patients. The discussion about the use of hormone therapy takes oodles of time. I spend a solid hour with every one of my new patients and at least forty-five minutes with repeat customers. After we come up with a plan of action together, I ask my patients to check in with me by e-mail or phone after three months (or sooner if they need me) to discuss what is improving and what still needs tweaking. I have such a passion for this field, I happily spend evening and weekend hours sorting issues out. The practice of midlife women's health is very time intensive.

When it comes to your multitude of treatment choices, remember that we all have to start somewhere. But we do not necessarily have to end there. Time will tell. If you still have symptoms that need to be addressed after starting hormone therapy, blood levels will not guide you. Only you and your symptoms can show us the way home.

I AM WOMAN, HEAR ME ROAR!

It will come as no surprise to you that some of my patients are curious to know what I have chosen for my own midlife journey. If you ever meet me in person, you might notice my high level of energy and overall good humor. Perhaps you will be more interested in my youthful skin or full head of hair, lightly sprinkled with just a few well-earned grays. My secret to health and wellness started in my late twenties when I made a commitment to regular exercise, healthy eating (mostly), and absolutely never smoking! After I experienced my first earth-shattering hot flash at the age of forty-five, along with night sweats, poor sleep, irritability, and brain fog, I made the decision to start a continuous low-dose birth control pill. I was feeling better within a month. I plan to continue this strategy until I am fifty-five. After that, when I officially join the Menopause Club, I will start hormone therapy immediately.

I would like to reveal another secret to you. I have decided that I would like to live until the age of eighty-five. I have specifically chosen that age because I feel confident that I can get there with enough health and wealth to enjoy myself and not be a burden to anyone. However, I retain the right to renegotiate that number when I hit eighty-four.

MENOPAUSE TREATMENT WRAP-UP

It is important for you to know that the best choice for one woman is not necessarily going to be the best choice for the next one. And let's not forget that perimenopause is different from menopause, and that natural menopause is different from surgical menopause. Therefore, you really do have to weigh all the available treatment choices and also find the right healthcare professional to help you on your own journey.

By the way, you might be wondering why I didn't list the names of all the current hormone therapy options available on the market today. It's not like I don't know them. And I do realize that you want me to name names. The truth is that by the time my book hits the shelves, some of today's choices will be gone and replaced by the newest kids on the block. Out with the old and in with the new. My not-so-secret wish is that *Menopause Confidential* will remain relevant, informative, and helpful to midlife women for many, many years to come.

The great and powerful Wizard of Oz . . . I mean Dr. Tara Allmen . . . has spoken.

CHAPTER 17

I Want to Feel Like a Natural Woman

There must be something to acupuncture . . .
you never see any sick porcupines.

—BOB GODDARD

As YOU KNOW, 80 percent of women will experience uncomfortable hot flashes for longer than ten years. Naturally, you may be inclined to try an over-the-counter solution first, because that feels safer and easier. It usually takes only a few months of suffering before you march off to the nearest health food vitamin store and pick up several bottles of different menopause remedies. In fact, 50 to 80 percent of midlife women use nonhormonal therapies to treat their menopausal symptoms, such as hot flashes, night sweats, and all the rest. Most women choose these products based on what the packaging says or what the young salesperson recommends as the most popular. If you can name a symptom, there's a product on the shelf that promises to cure it. The truth of the matter is that much of what's out there is a waste of your valuable time and hard earned money.

So how are you supposed to know what works? Should you eat more soy, take Chinese herbs, try black cohosh, explore the use of acupuncture, or sign up for yoga? If those choices are of interest to you, how long should you stick with them before you decide whether they are helping enough or not at all? Which vitamins and supplements should midlife women really try? Do fish oil capsules and vitamin E do anything?

Of course, the first person you should consult is your health-care professional rather than a sales clerk. However, the reality is that many in my profession are not knowledgeable about all of the alternative options available to treat menopause symptoms. I come to this conversation from a different perspective. Although I was born and raised in New York City, I completed my OB-GYN residency training in San Francisco, a city that truly embraces the use of complementary and alternative medicine. So while I will always be a daughter of New York, I feel that I am also a sister of San Francisco. There are definitely some good nonmedical approaches you can try for symptom relief.

SHOW ME THE EVIDENCE

The North American Menopause Society recently came out with a position statement on nonhormonal management of hot flashes and night sweats. Both clinical and research experts in this field reviewed all of the available scientific literature to create an evidence-based document to help us understand what really works well and what is simply a bunch of baloney. Now, I enjoy a delicious Oscar Mayer bologna sandwich as much as the next gal, especially when I slather on my favorite Hellmann's mayonnaise. However, as you have already learned in chapter 12, "Hooray for Colonoscopy!," we really should try to avoid processed meat. So let me cut through all the baloney and get right to the real meat of the matter. (Have I managed to turn off all of my vegetarian readers?)

Some of you are going to get mad at me for excluding approaches that both you and your best friend have tried and absolutely swear have cured your hot flashes and night sweats. In my experience, so many of these remedies work for a period of time. Then, lo and behold, the symptoms return with a vengeance. I know this first-hand, because that is when you show up at my office lugging a bag full of half-empty bottles. The point of this chapter is to help you choose effective alternative therapies that have some good science to back them up. No woman I know has extra time or money to waste.

NONPRESCRIPTION THERAPIES THAT WORK (BUT SOMETIMES DON'T)

Weight loss in overweight and obese women has definitely been shown to improve menopause symptoms. Of course, the tricky part is to figure out how to lose weight. I revealed the secret to weight loss in chapter 7, "What's the Skinny on Weight Gain?"

Cognitive behavioral therapy (CBT) is a short-term goal-oriented psychotherapy offered by a trained mental health professional. It can help you change negative thought patterns and learn effective ways to deal with challenging situations. CBT strategies that have been studied for menopausal symptoms include the daily practice of relaxation *combined* with paced breathing and good sleep hygiene.

Mindfulness-based stress reduction (MBSR) uses mindfulness meditation in conjunction with yoga to help handle stress. You are taught to approach thoughts, feelings, and sensations in a non-reactive way and to focus on the present moment, letting anxiety-provoking thoughts of the past or future slip away. This reduction in stress subsequently leads to a diminished intensity of hot flashes.

Clinical hypnosis is a mind-body therapy taught by a trained clinician. It is designed to facilitate a deeply relaxed state by utilizing individualized mental imagery and the power of suggestion. It is effective in improving mood and sleep as well as reducing hot flashes. For it to work, you have to be able to get into a deeply relaxed state. That automatically excludes me!

Stellate ganglion block (SGB) is a technique using local anesthesia injected into your cervical spine. It is not clear how or why it works, but it does indeed reduce hot flashes.

NONPRESCRIPTION THERAPIES THAT DON'T WORK (BUT SOMETIMES DO)

Black cohosh is the most commonly purchased botanical for the treatment of menopausal symptoms. It's been around for decades. The active ingredients are unknown, and the mechanism of action is unclear. Black cohosh really doesn't work any better than a placebo, which means that 30 percent of you will get some relief for some period of time. And there are some definite safety concerns involving the liver. As an aside, my husband always jokes that I should fill up a bottle with placebo pills and label it "Dr. Allmen's Menopause Miracle Cure." The placebo effect is very impressive!

Soy foods and supplements are a popular choice to help relieve hot flashes. I participated in an extensive yearlong review of all the available scientific literature that ultimately resulted in the 2011 North American Menopause Society position statement on the role of soy products in menopausal health. It turns out that *only* about 30 percent of U.S. women can metabolize soy foods and supplements in a way that allows them to utilize the specific soy metabolite known as S-equol, which likely helps relieve hot flashes. Soy foods are healthy and delicious. Enjoy them. However, do not depend on them for symptom relief.

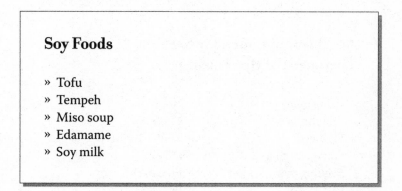

Soy Foods

» Tofu
» Tempeh
» Miso soup
» Edamame
» Soy milk

Acupuncture is a traditional component of Chinese medicine in which needles are inserted into the skin at specific points of the body. The scientific studies to date do not support the use of acupuncture for the treatment of hot flashes. That does not mean it can't be useful in other areas. As a physician, I have had only one experience with acupuncture. Years ago, my pregnant patient arrived at Labor and Delivery with her acupuncturist. She respectfully asked me if it was all right to have acupuncture needles placed on her body to help with labor pain. I was not familiar with the practice, but I went along anyway. Much to my surprise, my patient had one of the most comfortable birth experiences I have ever witnessed. When it was time to deliver the placenta, I was again asked if it was okay to place more needles. By this time, I was a believer!

Chiropractic intervention is not recommended for the treatment of hot flashes, because no clinical trials have been done.

Yoga does not help reduce hot flashes. To all of you yoginis out there, please do not get into the Warrior Pose. Downward, Dog! However, I have peeked into many yoga classes while on my way to spin class. Yoga looks very hard, and everyone seems to be in great shape. I plan to sign up for yoga this year.

Not Recommended for the Treatment of Hot Flashes

- » Dong quai
- » St. John's wort
- » Flaxseed
- » Ginkgo biloba
- » Evening primrose oil
- » Red clover
- » Wild yam
- » Ginseng
- » Hops
- » Maca
- » Rhubarb extract
- » Omega-3 fatty acids
- » Pine bark
- » Pollen extract
- » Fish oil capsules
- » Vitamin E

TIME IS UP

I would like to end this chapter with my philosophy on alternative treatments for menopausal symptoms. Even when science does not support the use of some interventions for the specific treatment of hot flashes, there may still be a place for them to help with other aspects of our health and wellness. If you want to try eating grapefruits while standing on your head, I will support you. Although I might giggle a little bit. There is definitely not one right answer or a one-size-fits-all approach to midlife women's health. However, based on all of the scientific evidence to date, limit your exploration of any one strategy to three months. If black cohosh has not worked for you by then, it is never going to work for you. Ever.

Now who can advise me on which yoga class to try first?

CHAPTER 18

Do I Really Have to Lift Weights Too?

My grandmother started walking five miles a
day when she was sixty. She's ninety-seven now,
and we don't know where the heck she is.

—ELLEN DEGENERES

FOR MY GENERATION, THE concept of aerobic exercise really came
together after Jane Fonda released her famous 1980s exercise video.
I can still hear Jane telling us to "feel the burn" as we squatted in
unison to achieve firmer bottoms. Jane *still* looks fitter than most
of us. I also fondly remember the step class that I took twice a week
when I lived in San Francisco. I was the annoying exercise enthusi-
ast who got to class early so I could get a spot in the front row. You
know the type. I practically never lifted a weight, though. It just
wasn't that much fun.

However, reaching midlife becomes an exercise game changer for most of us. As you have already learned in chapter 7, "What's the Skinny on Weight Gain?," you are redistributing body fat to your middle and losing valuable muscle mass. Since muscle is much more efficient at burning calories, it behooves us to maintain what we've got left. When we finally and begrudgingly come to the realization that we cannot fit into our favorite clothes despite eating well and continuing with our usual three-days-a-week aerobics class, something's gotta give. That something, as it turns out, is strength training.

The secret to *safe* strength training in midlife is to use light weights. By that, I mean weights that are no more than 5 to 10 pounds. Now I know that a few serious weight lifters among you are going to disagree with me regarding this puny poundage. But remember, the goal for midlifers is health and wellness. Women should strive to maximize their strength training while being careful to avoid injury. I totally disagree with the old saying "No pain, no gain." If you are experiencing pain when you lift weights, something did indeed give.

IT'S ALWAYS GOOD TO REVIEW

The Department of Health and Human Services (HHS) recommends both aerobic activity and strength training. And the American Heart Association (AHA) has laid it all out nicely for us, as described in chapter 7, "What's the Skinny on Weight Gain?," and chapter 15, "I Left My Heart in San Francisco." However, since many midlife women suffer from brain fog and poor memory, I will review the guidelines once again.

When it comes to heart health, you must engage in at least 150 minutes of moderate aerobic activity or 75 minutes of vigorous aerobic activity every week. Remember that what is good for the heart is also good for the brain. As for help with weight loss, you will have to increase your regimen to 60 minutes every single day. The recommendation for strength training is twice a week for at least 30 minutes.

Get Moving!

Heart and overall good health: 150 minutes of moderate aerobic activity or 75 minutes of vigorous aerobic activity weekly

Weight loss: 60 minutes of moderate aerobic activity daily

Muscle maintenance: 30 minutes of strength training twice weekly

---

All physical activity counts toward our health and wellness goals. So keep on dancing, gardening, swimming, and biking, if hitting the gym is not your thing. I just went skiing this weekend. Look out, Lindsey Vonn!

As for all of you die-hard runners, it's much better to switch over to fast walking and avoid injury to your knees and lower back. I get a lot of resistance when I offer up this advice. All I can say is I have never met a midlife runner who has not ultimately succumbed to injury. Poor knees.

WHAT IS THE BEST EXERCISE FOR BONE HEALTH?

Like everything else, when it comes to bones, you've got to use them or lose them. An exercise program aimed at improving bone health should specifically target posture, balance, gait, coordination, and hip and trunk stabilization rather than general aerobic exercise.

As you have learned in chapter 14, "Sticks and Stones Can Break Your Bones," the menopause transition is a time of rapid bone loss. For years, midlife women have been encouraged to lift weights in order to increase bone density and reduce the risk of bone fracture. As it turns out, the scientific evidence does not show that this actually happens. Strength training during midlife does not correlate with a significant increase in bone mass and a reduced fracture risk. I know this is shocking news to those of you with bone loss, since you have been told otherwise. However, weight training does increase muscle mass, which plays an important role in improving balance and overall strength. That will translate into less falling down, which will subsequently result in fewer fractures.

So let me be perfectly clear on the issue of menopause and bone health. I know that after reading "Sticks and Stones Can Break Your Bones" you are now eating enough calcium and vitamin D. However, for those of you who are at higher risk for osteoporosis, you really should consider the use of hormone therapy or a bisphosphonate to prevent the inevitable rapid bone loss that occurs at menopause. Strength training and calcium just won't cut the mustard for bone building when it comes to this specific time period.

ACHIEVING BALANCE

The secret to reducing the risk of bone fracture in midlife really lies in balance training. The scientific studies have focused on the regular practice of Tai Chi, with its flowing movements and poses. But many activities that strengthen your core and improve lower-body strength will do the job. Yoga definitely enhances balance. So does ballroom dancing, especially for all of you waltzers and fox-trotters. But don't fret if you do not have an Arthur Murray Dance Studio nearby. You can become less wobbly right in your own home. Just practice standing on one leg like a stork, while pressing your other leg against the first one. Make sure you are next to a wall, in case you start to topple over. Hold that position for as long as you can. Then switch legs. And if you really want to become an expert balancer, assume your stork position with your eyes closed.

As you recall from "Sticks and Stones Can Break Your Bones," the number one cause of fracture is falling down. So work on your balance, and do not fall down.

GET YOUR CHILDREN MOVING!

The secret to achieving lifelong bone health starts with regular physical activity in childhood. Regarding the formative bone building tween and teen years, the scientific evidence clearly demonstrates that kids who engage in daily walking, running, and jumping show up to adulthood with higher peak bone mass. When kids stop being physically active, they lose all that bone benefit over time. So whether it is basketball, tennis, soccer, or hopscotch, we really do need to continue schlepping our kids hither and thither to help them achieve their best bone potential. I just signed my daughter up for a gymnastics class, and I take my son to hip-hop dance. Good mommy.

That reminds me of a childhood memory, when Nana used to yell at my brother and me for jumping on her bed. I wish I had known then what I know now! So get your kids off their iPads and out to the playground or park for a rousing game of tag. And by "your kids," I also mean my own.

MY EXERCISE GLORY DAYS

I have always loved the camaraderie of an aerobic exercise class. There is something really supportive about having other women around, suffering loudly and succeeding proudly, together. For me, the best part of my aerobics workout was always the mental health benefits. After every Barry's Bootcamp, there was no challenge I could not handle. And then I hit my forties. That's when my children came along and all my extra time went away. That is also when I joined the symptomatic Perimenopause Club.

Instead of giving up on exercise completely, I made a few changes to accommodate my new and even busier life. I dropped the expensive Equinox membership, complete with steam room and fluffy towels. And then I bought a zoo. That's just an expression I use when I purchase something that is big and costly. What I actually bought was a treadmill.

The secret to using your new treadmill is to install a TV in front of it. I walk briskly on a slight incline, as if I am hiking up a hill. To help pass the time, I either watch TV or phone every person I know. I carry 3- to 5-pound weights, alternating biceps and triceps curls, in order to combine strength training with more intense cardio. I always commit to a minimum of thirty minutes. On some days, that's all the time I have. When I need some inspiration to push me to forty-five minutes or longer, I pull out my secret weapon . . . my fiftieth-birthday disco music playlist. No one gets me movin' and groovin' more than the Bee Gees and Michael Jackson.

As for my proclamation in chapter 17, "I Want to Feel like a Natural Woman," I will indeed sign up this summer for my very first yoga class. That is when my kids head off to camp, and I will have no more excuses left.

THE BEST IS YET TO COME

As a fifty-something, I am more committed to my own health and wellness than ever before. And though my time, energy, and enthusiasm for exercise have evolved over the years, I am smarter now. And so are you. We just have to figure out what physical activity, both aerobic and strength training, we can achieve safely and forevermore, until death do us part.

I would like to give a shout-out to all the hardworking women who are stuck in the Too Busy Bodies boat. Please join me. It's time to Rock the Boat. *Namaste.*

CHAPTER 19

The Top Five Studies That Rocked Women's Health

If we knew what it was we were doing, it would not be called research, would it?

—ALBERT EINSTEIN

THE WHOLE IDEA BEHIND this chapter came to me in the middle of the night, when I was having either a lovely dream or a terrible nightmare about writing a book. I suppose I should add *becoming a first-time author* to my personal list of sleep-disruption issues. Anyway, as a physician, I find it very unsettling that women mostly hear bad bits and pieces on the news about studies that affect major health issues, causing more confusion and worry than necessary. So it seemed like a swell idea to provide you with some brief summaries of my favorite women's health studies to help you really understand all the hubbub. Remember that knowledge is power. Prepare to rule the world . . . or at least manage the Internet hype.

As an aside, I now listen to every medical news report and read every scientific newspaper article with a cynical ear and a critical eye, suspicious that some reporter or writer may have a secret duty to sensationalize scary information and minimize good news, no matter what the topic.

THE NURSES' HEALTH STUDY (NHS), 1976 TO TODAY

This groundbreaking study falls into the category of observational, which means that researchers follow real women over time to see if there is a relationship between their medical and lifestyle practices and their various health issues. Observational studies cannot confirm an actual cause and effect. However, they can point a strong finger in one direction or another. An interesting example of this type of study is the association that was made after observing people who smoked cigarettes and their subsequent development of lung cancer. By now, you know how I feel about cigarette smoking.

The NHS is actually a series of observational studies that are still ongoing today. The first one was established in 1976 to investigate the long-term consequences of using birth control pills. Over the years, several hundred thousand nurses from around the country have been recruited to fill out questionnaires about their personal exposure to cigarette smoking, alcohol use, diet, physical activity, obesity, birth control pill use, and hormone therapy use. These same nurses have to fill out follow-up questionnaires every few years.

We owe these nurses a debt of gratitude. As a result of their efforts, researchers have made many important observations regarding women's health. As I always say to anyone who is scheduled for surgery or is admitted to a hospital, "Be nice to your nurses."

The following are the most important observations that have come from the NHS:

- Smoking cigarettes is associated with an increased risk of heart disease, stroke, colon cancer, hip fracture, and cataracts.

- A diet higher in red meat is associated with an increased risk of colon and premenopausal breast cancer.

- A Mediterranean-type diet reduces the risk of heart disease and stroke.

- Higher vitamin D and calcium supplement intake reduces the risk of colon cancer and hip fracture.

- Vegetables, especially green leafy ones, reduce the risk of impairments in memory and mental function.

- Physical activity of greater than three hours per week is associated with a decreased risk of heart disease and stroke, breast and colon cancer, hip fracture, and memory and mental-function impairment.

- Obesity is associated with an increased risk of postmenopausal breast cancer, heart disease, stroke, colon cancer, and cataracts. Interestingly, the extra fat padding around hips seems to be protective against hip fracture.

- Alcohol use is associated with an increased risk of breast and colon cancer as well as hip fracture. On the fun flip side, moderate alcohol use is also associated with a reduced risk of heart disease and memory and mental-function impairment.

- Current birth control pill use is associated with an increased risk of breast cancer, heart disease, and stroke but a reduced risk of colon cancer.

  Remember that observational studies do not demonstrate cause and effect. As far as the breast cancer issue is concerned, birth control pills are associated with women getting annual visits in order to get their prescriptions. That leads to more breast cancer surveillance. When you look for something, you might actually find it.

- Hormone therapy used for longer than five years is associated with an increased risk of breast cancer and stroke and a reduced risk of colon cancer and hip fracture. When started early in menopause, it is also associated with a reduced risk of heart disease.

  Again, I must remind you that observational studies do not demonstrate cause and effect. I know that many of you are having a hard time understanding the association between hormone therapy and breast cancer. Please review chapter 11, "It's All About the Breast," and chapter 16, "Potions, Patches, and Pills, Oh My!" You will be glad you did.

You could say that the Nurses' Health Study is the mother of all women's health studies. A lot of what we know today has come out of this far-reaching research depot. And as a direct result of this provocative observational data, randomized controlled trials have been designed to kick the level of scientific research in women's health up a few notches.

THE POSTMENOPAUSAL ESTROGEN/PROGESTIN INTERVENTIONS STUDY (PEPI), 1987 TO 1990

PEPI is a randomized controlled trial (RCT), which is considered to be the gold standard of scientific research. It is designed to study people who have been randomly assigned to different treatment groups. Then these people are followed to see how they respond to the particular intervention. An example of this kind of study could be a silly version of *The Biggest Loser*, where one group is assigned a healthy diet and daily exercise regimen while the other group sits in front of a TV all day, eating bonbons and watching the show. The weight-loss and health-gain results would clearly be greater in the first group and attributable to their healthy lifestyle choices.

PEPI is a fun word to say and makes me feel all the more peppy to explain the results of this important study to you. It evaluated over 800 healthy women, ages forty-five to sixty-four, to learn about the risks and benefits of various hormone therapy regimens on heart disease and bone health.

The following is the most important information gleaned from PEPI:

- Women with a uterus taking systemic estrogen therapy must also take progesterone to protect the uterine lining from abnormal growth called hyperplasia and cancer.

- Hormone therapy increases bone mineral density in the hip and spine.

- Hormone therapy increases breast density on mammographic screening.

- Hormone therapy does not cause weight gain.

- Hormone therapy lowers the risk of heart disease by increasing good HDL cholesterol and decreasing bad LDL cholesterol.

It was this last bit of information that caused the most excitement in the women's health community, because it supported the observation seen in the NHS that estrogen protects women against heart disease.

THE STUDY OF WOMEN'S HEALTH ACROSS THE NATION (SWAN), 1996 TO TODAY

SWAN is an observational study designed to characterize the physiological and psychological changes that occur during the transition from perimenopause to menopause. Over 3,000 premenopausal women ranging in age from forty-two to fifty-two were enrolled. Researchers have been hard at work compiling comprehensive data that focus on midlife heart disease, bone health, depression, and cognitive function.

What makes SWAN particularly important is the fact that it recognizes the value of observing different ethnic backgrounds including Caucasian, African American, Japanese, Hispanic, and Chinese women. Ethnicity plays a big part in the menopause transition experience. Researchers are continuing to observe this group of women, now in menopause, as they journey toward their swan song.

The following is the most important information currently gathered from SWAN:

- African American and Hispanic women have the highest body mass index and experience hot flashes longer than Caucasian and Asian women do.

- Hot flashes can affect women for as long as fourteen years.

- African American women are more likely to undergo a hysterectomy and surgical menopause.

- Hispanic women are more likely to undergo early or premature natural menopause and develop metabolic syndrome and diabetes.

- Women who start flashing earlier in their transition will also flash for longer.

- Women with longer-lasting symptoms tend to have a lower socioeconomic status, less education, more perceived stress, and more depression and anxiety.

- Late perimenopause is associated with rapid bone loss and more sleep difficulty.

- Hot flashes and depression are associated with an increased risk of heart disease.

HEART AND ESTROGEN/PROGESTIN REPLACEMENT STUDY (HERS), 1998 TO 2002

HERS was the first large randomized controlled trial to examine the effect of hormone therapy on women who already had heart disease. The purpose of the study was to prove that hormone therapy protects against heart disease, which is what previous observational data had suggested. About 2,800 women with an average age of sixty-seven were randomly assigned to either get hormone therapy or a placebo. Researchers monitored them for four years.

The following is the most important information learned from HERS:

- Hormone therapy does not prevent future heart attacks or death from heart issues in women who already have established heart disease.

- Hormone therapy increases the risk of blood clots in veins and lungs.

- Hormone therapy increases the risk of gallbladder disease.

- Hormone therapy increases good HDL cholesterol and decreases bad LDL cholesterol.

- Women who are more than ten years past their last menstrual cycle should not start hormone therapy for the prevention of heart disease or recurrent heart attacks.

- Women who have already started hormone therapy at the time of menopause for the treatment of symptoms do not need to discontinue because of this study.

THE WOMEN'S HEALTH INITIATIVE (WHI), 1993 TO 2007 (WITH A PIT STOP IN 2002)

WHI is the King Kong of all confusing and misunderstood women's health studies and likely the only one you have heard about. When part of the study was stopped in 2002, it made the news big-time. All the hoopla still reverberates to this day. The initial results from WHI were reported in 2002, causing a generation of women to stop using hormone therapy. Whether you realize it or not, the WHI is the reason so many of you are frightened to start therapy. But like most things in life, once you understand the issue better, the world is less scary. Let me introduce you to my friend, King Kong.

The Women's Health Initiative was a randomized controlled trial designed to examine the effects of hormone therapy on heart attacks; stroke; blood clots; bone fractures; breast, colon, and uterine cancer; and overall causes of death. One could argue that King

Kong bit off more than he could chew. WHI surpassed HERS in terms of size, duration, and goals. Over 27,000 healthy women ages fifty to seventy-nine were enrolled in the hormone therapy arms of the trial, with the intention of studying them for ten years.

Healthy women without a uterus on estrogen-only therapy were studied for over eight years. Healthy women who had a uterus and were therefore on both estrogen and synthetic progesterone therapy were studied for five years. The trials were stopped early when a concerning breast cancer and heart attack trend was observed. Once the initial alarm sounded in 2002, specifically for the women taking both estrogen and synthetic progesterone, everyone in the village began to panic. That's when all the townspeople came out to kill King Kong.

The following is the most important information currently derived from the WHI:

- Risks and benefits of hormone therapy depend a lot on the age you are when you join the Menopause Club, when you start hormone therapy, which treatment you choose, whether you have a uterus, and how long you continue using hormones.

- Hormone therapy should be used for the treatment of menopause symptoms, vaginal dryness, and the prevention of bone fractures.

- The best candidates for hormone therapy are healthy women who are suffering from menopause symptoms, less than ten years from their last menstrual period, and under the age of sixty when they start.

- Hormone therapy should not be used for the prevention of heart disease if you already have established heart disease, are more than ten years from your last menstrual cycle, or are over the age of sixty.

- Hormone therapy is associated with a reduced risk of hip and spine fracture and colon cancer.

- Hormone therapy is associated with an increased risk of blood clots, stroke, heart attacks, and gallbladder disease.

- Hormone therapy in women with a uterus is associated with a modest increased risk in breast cancer when used for longer than five years.

- On the fun flip side, younger women without a uterus who use estrogen-only therapy seem to have a decreased risk of breast cancer, heart disease, diabetes, stroke, bone fracture, and death.

If you are a healthy woman under the age of sixty or less than ten years from your last menstrual cycle, the wonderful wizarding world of hormone therapy is yours to explore. All the risks that you have heard and read about generally do not apply to you. That is especially true for women who do *not* have a uterus and therefore do *not* need to take progesterone.

This is how I like to explain risk to my *healthy* menopausal women who are considering the use of hormone therapy. No matter which risk you choose from the laundry list, the likelihood that it will happen to you is very small and similar to the risk of getting a date with George Clooney. I hope that sets your mind at ease regarding risk.

BONUS STUDIES

I probably should reveal that the original title of this chapter was "The Top Ten Studies That Rocked Women's Health." However, after covering five of them, I decided that some of you might be getting a wee bit overwhelmed or just outright bored. I want *Menopause Confidential* to inform you without causing head-spinning dizziness or yawning.

So it is with your very best interest in mind that I just lightly mention some other studies out there that have continued the important dialogue on midlife women's health. Just head over to The Google to learn about the Kronos Early Estrogen Prevention Study (KEEPS) with its key findings that hormone therapy started early in your transition improves mood, memory, heart health, and bone density. And while you are surfing the Internet, you might as well catch the wave called Early Versus Late Intervention Trial with Estradiol (ELITE), which supports the timing hypothesis that hormone therapy started earlier in menopause is heart-helpful.

ANOTHER SECRET REVEALED

Now I will venture where no book on midlife women's health has gone before and reveal the significant and sad consequences that occurred when women did not receive accurate and well-explained information over a decade ago. Because of the WHI, many women abruptly discontinued hormone therapy, and many more decided not to try it at all. This reality provided a research opportunity to study the health effects of stopping hormone therapy or avoiding it altogether. The results continue to come in, and they are disheartening. As it turns out, the generation of women caught in the cross fire of WHI are having more heart and bone attacks and dying earlier in life than the women who braved the hormone therapy firestorm and stayed the course. So while we cannot be "Forever Young," we can most certainly be Healthy for a Lot Longer when we have access to the best scientific research explained in the least confusing way.

THE SCIENCE WRAP-UP

What you should take away from all the scientific literature to date is that midlife presents a unique time to change your health destiny. From improving your lifestyle choices to considering the use of hormone therapy, you are at an exciting crossroads. Take advantage of this marvelous stained-glass window of opportunity. And lead the way for the next generation. Since it is much easier for most of us to walk through a wide open door than to squeeze through a tiny window, encourage all of your forty-something friends to get started on their quest for the best information available. Don't show up to menopause clueless. You can help the cause by letting your friends in on the secret of *Menopause Confidential*.

CHAPTER 20

Every Man Needs a Gynecologist

Marriage is a relationship in which one person
is always right and the other is the husband.

—ANONYMOUS

WHENEVER MEN ASK ME what I do for a living, I tell them that I am
a physician. I never tell them right away that I am a gynecologist
because, when I do, it shuts down the conversation faster than you
can say "gynecologist." That word seems to make men squirm with
discomfort. Some have tried valiantly to respond with a witty come-
back. Most men just look down at their shoes in bewilderment. It is
all very awkward.

So I developed a strategy to put men at ease. Right after I say the
word "gynecologist," I launch right into why every man needs one.
Men become immediately intrigued and give me their full attention.

Now I will share the secret with you. The reason every man needs a gynecologist is because every man has a grandmother, mother, aunt, sister, girlfriend, wife, or daughter. It is my job to keep all of those women healthy. And if I do my job well, every man will be much happier. You are all welcome, men of the world.

> Most men do not know what to do when the change happens. I still don't, but I am happier now that my wife has figured things out.
>
> —MIKE L.

I always chuckle at the expression "Happy wife, happy life." It is especially true for those men who are married to women going through perimenopause and menopause. I hear about it from both sides of the conversation. The men say to me, "My wife is crazy. Can you help her?" The women say . . . well, I do not want to reveal what the women say! However, most women seem to have the exact same complaints about their menfolk, which has led me to the conclusion that we are all married to the same guy.

My husband is one of the luckiest fellas in the land to actually be *married* to a gynecologist. Rest assured that I tell him so about once a week. I have saved him a lot of time and money by knowing exactly what to do when I have personally experienced a yeast infection, PMS, childbirth, and perimenopausal symptoms. He got to skip out on Lamaze classes, OB visits, and breastfeeding tutorials. When it was time to go to Labor and Delivery for our first child, my husband had both a cold and a hacking cough. So I quarantined him in one corner of the room. I can still remember the smell of his

Halls cherry lozenges permeating my birth experience. And when it was time to deliver our second child, I left my husband home for a few extra hours as I headed off to the hospital. No need for both of us to have to wait around. I even sent him home early that first night after I gave birth, so he could get a good rest. There are many perks to being married to a gynecologist!

> Despite the fact that I am married to a gynecologist and an expert in midlife women's health, I will still have to read *Menopause Confidential*, because I have no idea what my wife is talking about half the time.
>
> —DR. ALLMEN'S HUSBAND

Here is another expression that I also love and would like to share with you. After I got married and started having the kind of squabbles that married people do, my friend offered up that old adage "Do you want to be right, or do you want to be married?" All relationships are a challenge. Communication and kindness are especially necessary when women start that long march into madness . . . I mean, menopause. This is where we need to take charge of helping the menfolk understand our particular needs. As you can see by the quotes scattered throughout this chapter, from the husbands of my very own patients, the fellas really need our help.

Men don't get one single lecture on midlife women's health anywhere. Frankly, most women never get a lecture either. The difference, however, is that our symptoms quickly lead us to seek information and solutions. Again, men just wind up looking down at their shoes in bewilderment.

In my experience, most men would like just a little enlightenment on this topic, so that they can learn how to be more supportive and understanding when women start hot-flashing and hell-raising all over the place. I am always delighted when men join their women at my office for the discussion. As I already revealed in chapter 3, "My Husband Thinks I'm Crazy," I have called many a man on the phone to reassure him that his gal is indeed sane and that help is on the way.

> I don't know if I am allowed to say this, but our once happy marriage took a turn for the worse after menopause. Now that my wife is starting to feel better, we are slowly rebuilding our connection.
>
> —JOHN D.

Right now, your man only knows what he sees. You are not the "hot!" woman he fell in love with all those years ago! You are just hot. And moody, sweaty, mad as a hatter, disinterested in sex, and becoming slightly obsessed with the air-conditioning controls. He does not know about all the things going on beneath the surface that are causing hot flash havoc. So it is your job to see that he gets educated.

> Once my wife started using hormone therapy, the heavens parted and the angels began to sing.
>
> —DAVID K.

MEN ARE PEOPLE TOO

If you are a man who is, possibly, being forced at this very moment to read *Menopause Confidential*, I want you to know how much I appreciate your side of the story. You have shaped the way I think about my role as a physician in the field of midlife women's health and wellness. Your opinion matters, and your voice should be heard. So I encourage you to speak up and ask questions. Make your feelings known. Tag along to office visits to show your support. You will definitely learn something. Besides, I want you there. In all the years that I have been caring for women, I am happiest when I see that they have dragged their men along for the ride. As you now know, every man needs a gynecologist!

> I insisted that I go with my wife to her doctor's appointment. I wanted to make sure she told the whole truth, because I was miserable too. It was very helpful for both of us.
>
> —SHELDON H.

THE QUESTION BEGETS A QUESTION

After many years of marriage, I would finally like to respond to my friend regarding the old expression about being right versus being married. My dad used to say to me, "I don't like to say I told you so. I *love* to say I told you so!" He also used to proclaim, "I am the big boss . . . but your mother is the real boss." He was a very funny fellow. And just like my dad, I prefer to be right. But now I would like to pose the following question to all of you. Why can't women be both?

For more information on this topic, someone will need to create a website called Men-o'-PauseConfidential.com to share men secrets with women!

CHAPTER 21

Your Story

But enough about me. Let's talk about
you . . . what do you think of me?

—BETTE MIDLER IN THE MOVIE *BEACHES*

WHEN I STARTED WRITING *Menopause Confidential*, I thought it
was important for you to know *my* story. Not only did I want you
to learn about my qualifications and credentials to write a book
on midlife women's health, but I also wanted to convey my own
experience with this very personal journey. My thoughts, feelings,
hopes, and dreams about embarking on this final frontier are, in
many ways, just like yours. And like you, I also have fears about
the future. At this point in my life, though, mine mostly pertain to
making sure I raise healthy, happy, and productive children. I would
like one of them to grow up to become the president of the United

States of America, because my husband is a political news junkie. And I'd like the other one to run a major motion picture studio, so I can go to the Oscars. I'll let you know how that works out. But the one thing I don't have to worry about is how I am going to manage my own midlife health and wellness. I've got that covered. And now, after reading my book, you do too!

Women experience perimenopause and menopause in many different ways. A few lucky ducks are going to be able to swim right through the change of life without so much as a peep. The rest of us are going to have to deal with a variety of challenging symptoms that may make us feel like we are drowning. But *Menopause Confidential* is your *life preserver*. There is no one-size-fits-all approach to good midlife health. But that is nothing to worry about, because now you have all the information necessary to discover what works *specifically* for you. Don't you feel better already?

By the way, I never set out to write a book. The most I had ever written before *Menopause Confidential* was a letter. Sometimes I like to joke that I am a doctor, and occasionally, I even play one on TV. But the opportunity to become an author hit me like a perfect storm, in a good way. And although writing a book is one of the hardest things I have ever done, it has all been worth it. I am absolutely tickled *pink* that I have been given a chance to calm the fears and quiet the anxieties that so many of you feel when that first hot flash strikes. I hope you are not only more relaxed, but also more confident that you will get through this whole midlife thing with style and grace. After all, you are now practically an expert on perimenopause and menopause. You have learned the anatomy of a hot flash, the secret to making sex enjoyable again, and how to get rid of that persistent urge to pee. You can rationally explain why you are acting so crazy. You know the secrets to weight loss, gorgeous skin, and restful sleep. And you are up-to-date on when to get a mammogram, Pap test, and colonoscopy. Finally, when it comes to symptom relief, you know what works, what doesn't, and what is a complete waste of time. So the next time you show up at your healthcare professional's office, I expect you to hold your head high and show off your newfound knowledge. Make me proud!

One of the things I love the most about my day job is when I get a call or an e-mail from a patient who says she left my office with a new lease on life. That does not mean that she changed everything in one day. It just means that she got started by walking home from work, choosing fish instead of a burger and fries, and throwing out the hot flash remedy she had been taking for six months without relief. That is all I ask of you. Start your journey to health by taking a baby step forward. All you have to do is put one foot in front of the other and soon you'll be walking out the door. In the words of the ancient Chinese philosopher Lao Tzu, "The journey of a thousand miles begins with a single step."

Although you may have originally picked up *Menopause Confidential* with its come-hither title and pretty pink color to learn all the secrets to cooling down hot flashes, heating up sex drive, and taking back your once happy life, I hope you have found the information valuable in helping you develop a real health game plan for the future. Don't forget that menopause marks the beginning of even more challenges like heart disease, osteoporosis, diabetes, Alzheimer's disease, and cancer. So this is your call to action! Seize the moment to take charge of your health, and you will become the richest person in the entire world. The heck with the Powerball.

Believe me when I say that *Menopause Confidential* is also going to help you come to terms with aging. We cannot turn back the clock, but having energy, vitality, and good health to spare is all that really matters. I think that the most beautiful women are the ones who radiate confidence and generosity of spirit. I also love women who smile a lot. Let go of that frowny face. It will only lead to wrinkles. Focus on feeling strong and vibrant. Soon, you will be unabashedly shouting your age from the rooftops, just like I do. So go forth, all you fabulous, smart, capable, and knowledgeable women of the world. And when you are not feeling so fabulous? Duck back into this book. I will always be here for you!

IT'S YOUR TURN

Now the time has come for you to tell me your unique story. We are all going to bring something different to this conversation. I want you to feel comfortable and confident when you share your journey with me or your own healthcare professional. In fact, I want you to be loud and proud when it comes to talking about your midlife health and wellness.

So let's get this party started. I am listening. Who wants to go first?

For the best way to tell me *your* story, visit www.drallmen.com.

ACKNOWLEDGMENTS

MY JOURNEY AS AN author began at the tender age of forty-nine and a half.

That is when Bonnie Solow, president of Solow Literary Enterprises, based near San Francisco, sent me a very encouraging e-mail, completely out of the blue, suggesting that I write a book. My first reaction was, "Who is this chick?" I probably should have Googled her, but the truth is that I cannot find anything on the Internet. Not even milk. Don't judge me. So after several e-mails, phone calls, and a face-to-face meeting in San Francisco a few months later, I learned that Bonnie is a smart, savvy, successful literary agent who has represented many bestselling authors. We took a nice long walk down Market Street to the San Francisco Bay, and that was that. Since I was just about to turn fifty, I decided to write a book. Why not? I'll tell you why not! Because writing a book is just about the hardest thing I have ever done. So thank you, Bonnie, for giving me this unbelievable opportunity to become an author. I may never forgive you.

Now for those of you who have no idea how this process works, I will reveal the secrets. The next thing you have to do is write a proposal for your unwritten book. Naively, I thought that meant that I could take a single sheet of paper and write, "I propose to write a book about midlife women's health." Turns out, it really means that you have to know precisely what you are going to write about, summarize all the chapters you have not yet written, compare your proposed book to what is already out there, and elaborate on why your book is going to be the best thing since sliced bread. That's where the amazing Daryn Eller, MLIS, based in Venice, California, joined my narrative. She is actually a real writer who helped me find my writing voice. Daryn, I think of you as my personal Tinker Bell, generously sprinkling fairy dust all over my words.

The proposal is sent to many publishers, and that is when the courting begins. I interview them. They interview me. And if an author is lucky, there are several interested suitors. After an exciting bidding war, Gideon Weil of HarperOne, based in San Francisco, emerged as the victor. He was my biggest cheerleader and gave me the confidence that I could really write something that would change the landscape for women. Nine months later, my baby, *Menopause Confidential*, was born. With Gideon's guidance and expertise, my book could even become the new benchmark for midlife women's health. Those are Gideon's words, not mine.

As with any birth experience, one needs some assistance. My midwife, if you will, was Carolyn Develen, chief operating officer of the North American Menopause Society (NAMS). Whenever I needed to connect with an expert on a particular subject, I e-mailed Carolyn, whose response time was measurable in minutes. Carolyn, if you did not already know how invaluable you are to NAMS, I am telling you now.

Many writers hire a ghostwriter, and I would like to unequivocally state that I wrote practically every word of this book all by myself. In the beginning, however, I did march around proclaiming to no one in particular, "My kingdom for a ghostwriter!" I soon found my own writing style, but I needed help with research. That is when the incomparable Batya Swift Yasgur, MA, LMSW, joined my team. Not only did Batya help me find the latest guidelines and updated information on all things perimenopause and menopause, she also patiently listened to me read each chapter and offered very helpful suggestions. Batya, I would like to thank you for laughing at all of my jokes, even after you had heard them for the twelfth time.

Kristin Mehus-Roe from Girl Friday Productions stuck with me until the bitter end as I edited and re-edited my manuscript long after I was allowed to make changes.

Of course, no author stands a chance of getting her book to the people without the hard work and dedication of a marketing and PR team. So thank you to Lorrie Lee and Winnie Hart at TwinEngine, Suzy Ginsburg, president and CEO at Global Communications Works, and the entire team at HarperOne and Worthy Marketing Group.

Finally, I would like to acknowledge my attorney, Joseph Vitulli, Esq., who made sure that I properly crossed my t's and dotted my i's on all the confusing contracts that came my way. We have known each other since we were ten years old. Joseph, I can honestly say that as we cruise through our fifties and beyond, you have also become my most trusted adviser and best friend.

It takes a village to raise a doctor. I am proud to introduce you to my Village People.

John C. Arpels, MD

Gloria A. Bachmann, MD

David A. Baker, MD

John P. Bilezikian, MD

Patricia Calayag, MD

Alyssa Dweck, MD, NCMP

Murray A. Freedman, MD

Steven R. Goldstein, MD, NCMP

Henry M. Hess, MD, PhD, NCMP

Howard N. Hodis, MD

Hadine Joffe, MD

Risa Kagan, MD, NCMP

Michael Katz, MD

David M. Kaufman, MD

Andrew M. Kaunitz, MD, NCMP

Sheryl A. Kingsberg, PhD

Michael L. Krychman, MD

Lisa C. Larkin, MD, NCMP

James H. Liu, MD, NCMP

Pauline M. Maki, PhD

JoAnn E. Manson, MD, NCMP

Michael R. McClung, MD

Lila E. Nachtigall, MD, NCMP

Sharon J. Parish, MD, NCMP

JoAnn V. Pinkerton, MD, NCMP

David J. Portman, MD, NCMP

Philip M. Sarrel, MD

George F. Sawaya, MD

Isaac Schiff, MD

Freya Schnabel, MD

Jan L. Shifren, MD, NCMP

Chrisandra Shufelt, MD, NCMP

Lee P. Shulman, MD

James A. Simon, MD, NCMP

Claudio N. Soares, MD, PhD

Holly L. Thacker, MD, NCMP

Wulf H. Utian, MD, PhD

Michelle P. Warren, MD, NCMP

Michelle R. Yagoda, MD

WHO WANTS TO KEEP LEARNING?

CHAPTER 1: GIRLS ARE MADE OF SUGAR
AND SPICE AND EVERYTHING NICE . . . AND
THAT EVERYTHING NICE IS ESTROGEN

The North American Menopause Society
www.menopause.org

CHAPTER 2: I AM HOT!

The North American Menopause Society
www.menopause.org

CHAPTER 3: MY HUSBAND THINKS I'M CRAZY

Massachusetts General Hospital Center for Women's Mental Health
www.womensmentalhealth.org

CHAPTER 4: MENOFOG ROLLS IN, FOCUS ROLLS OUT

The North American Menopause Society
www.menopause.org

Massachusetts General Hospital Center for Women's Mental Health
www.womensmentalhealth.org

CHAPTER 5: THERE IS NO REST FOR THE WEARY

National Sleep Foundation
www.sleepfoundation.org

CHAPTER 6: THE VAGINA IS LIKE LAS VEGAS, *BABY*!

The North American Menopause Society
www.menopause.org

International Society for the Study of Women's Sexual Health
www.ISSWSH.org

Vaginismus
www.vaginismus.com

MiddlesexMD
http://middlesexmd.com

MedAmour
https://medamour.com

CHAPTER 7: WHAT'S THE SKINNY ON WEIGHT GAIN?

"Dietary Guidelines for Americans"
www.dietaryguidelines.gov

Weight Watchers
www.weightwatchers.com

United States Department of Agriculture
www.choosemyplate.gov

CHAPTER 8: TO PEE OR NOT TO PEE

Urology Care Foundation
www.urologyhealth.org

CHAPTER 9: WHO IS THAT WRINKLY OLD WOMAN IN THE MIRROR?

American Academy of Dermatology
www.aad.org

CHAPTER 10: FIFTY SHADES OF GRAY . . . HAIR

American Academy of Dermatology
www.aad.org

The Hair Foundation
www.hairfoundation.org

CHAPTER 11: IT'S ALL ABOUT THE BREAST

American Cancer Society
www.cancer.org

U.S. Preventive Services Task Force
www.uspreventiveservicestaskforce.org

The American College of Obstetricians and Gynecologists
www.acog.org

CHAPTER 12: HOORAY FOR COLONOSCOPY!

American Cancer Society
www.cancer.org/cancer

National Cancer Institute
www.cancer.gov

CHAPTER 13: THE LATEST RAP ABOUT THE PAP

Centers for Disease Control and Prevention (CDC)
www.cdc.gov/cancer/cervical/basic_info/screening.htm

CHAPTER 14: STICKS AND STONES
CAN BREAK YOUR BONES

The National Osteoporosis Foundation
www.nof.org

American Bone Health
www.americanbonehealth.org

NIH Osteoporosis and Related Bone Diseases National Resource Center
www.niams.nih.gov/health_Info/Bone

CHAPTER 15: I LEFT MY HEART IN SAN FRANCISCO

American Heart Association
www.heart.org

CHAPTER 16: POTIONS, PATCHES, AND PILLS, OH MY!

The North American Menopause Society
www.menopause.org

Advancing Health After Hysterectomy Foundation (AHAH)
http://www.empowher.com/hysterectomy/content/ahah
    -advancing-health-after-hysterectomy-foundation

CHAPTER 17: I WANT TO FEEL LIKE A NATURAL WOMAN

The North American Menopause Society
www.menopause.org

CHAPTER 18: DO I REALLY HAVE TO LIFT WEIGHTS TOO?

Centers for Disease Control and Prevention (CDC)
www.cdc.gov/physicalactivity/basics/older_adults/

Office of Disease Prevention and Health Promotion
health.gov/paguidelines/guidelines/chapter5.aspx

CHAPTER 19: THE TOP FIVE STUDIES
THAT ROCKED WOMEN'S HEALTH

Nurses' Health Study (NHS)
www.nhs3.org

National Heart, Lung, and Blood Institute (NHLBI)
www.nhlbi.nih.gov/news/press-releases/1998/the-hers-study
    -results-and-ongoing-studies-of-women-and-heart-disease

Study of Women's Health Across the Nation (SWAN)
www.swanstudy.org

Women's Health Initiative (WHI)
https://www.nhlbi.nih.gov/whi/whi_faq.htm

Harvard Health Publications

http://www.health.harvard.edu/womens-health/hormone-therapy
-the-next-chapter

CHAPTER 20: YOUR STORY

www.EmpowHER.com

www.drallmen.com

INDEX